Gastrointestinal Nursing

Gastrointestinal Nursing

Graeme D Smith
and
Roger Watson

Blackwell
Science

© 2005 by Blackwell Science Ltd, a Blackwell Publishing company

Editorial offices:
Blackwell Science Ltd, 9600 Garsington Road, Oxford OX4 2DQ, UK
    Tel: +44 (0) 1865 776868
Blackwell Publishing Inc., 350 Main Street, Malden, MA 02148–5020, USA
    Tel: +1 781 388 8250
Blackwell Science Asia Pty Ltd, 550 Swanston Street, Carlton, Victoria 3053,
Australia
    Tel: +61 (0)3 8359 1011

First published 2005

Library of Congress Cataloging-in-Publication Data
Smith, Graeme D.
    Gastrointestinal nursing / Graeme D. Smith and Roger Watson.
        p. ; cm.
    Includes bibliographical references and index.
    ISBN-13: 978-0-632-05294-3 (pbk. : alk. paper)
    ISBN-10: 0-632-05294-5 (pbk. : alk. paper)

1. Gastrointestinal system—Diseases—Nursing.
    [DNLM: 1. Gastrointestinal Diseases—nursing.   2. Digestive System.
WY 156.5 S648g 2005]   I. Watson, Roger, 1955–   II. Title.

    RC802.S615 2005
    616.3′3′0231—dc22
    2004024235

ISBN-10: 0-632-05294-5
ISBN-13: 978-0632-05294-3

A catalogue record for this title is available from the British Library

Set in 10/12.5pt Palatino
by Graphicraft Limited, Hong Kong
Printed and bound in India
by Replika Press Pvt Ltd, Kundli

For further information on Blackwell Publishing, visit our website:
www.blackwellnursing.com

Contents

Foreword

In 1991 I was presenter of the BBC's *Watchdog* programme, married to my co-presenter John Stapleton with a two-year-old son. Life was good. I had never heard of bowel cancer, had no idea that it was the second biggest cancer killer in the UK. So I had no worries that the subtle symptom I had spotted intermittently – just a bit of rectal bleeding – might be serious.

When my GP reassured me that it was 'nothing to worry about' at my age, 'probably piles', I believed him. It was a terrible shock to discover nearly a year later, through my persistence, that I had advanced bowel cancer, in the lymph nodes. Luckily I survived and have spent much of the last seven years working with leading colorectal specialist doctors and nurses on ways to save lives and improve quality of life for bowel cancer patients. I now appreciate how complex our insides are, and how difficult it can be to diagnose and treat digestive disorders. I also appreciate how vital well-trained, supportive nurses can be at every stage of the patient's journey.

I've learned a lot from reading this book and really recommend it to nurses with an interest in gastrointestinal diseases and conditions.

Lynn Faulds Wood
Bowel Cancer Campaign
Chairman of European Cancer Patient Coalition

Chapter 1
Introduction

Chapter objectives

After reading this chapter you should be able to:

- Understand the scope of nursing practice within the gastrointestinal setting.
- Describe the general responsibilities of the gastrointestinal nurse.
- Identify the specific role of the gastrointestinal nurse practitioners and nurse endoscopists.
- Relate the responsibilities of the nurse in the gastrointestinal setting to NMC policy.

Introduction

Over the last 20 years there have been many changes within the scope of practice in gastrointestinal nursing. In particular, the development of endoscopic equipment has resulted in the demand for skilled nurses not only to look after patients in this area but also to perform endoscopic procedures. Historically, nurses were required to attend patients whilst the doctor conducted the procedure.

This changed significantly in the United Kingdom with junior doctors' hours being reduced (http://www.doh.gov.uk/juniordoctors/ accessed 8 May 2004). The UKCC confirmed role extension in nursing with a timely document *The Scope of Professional Practice* in 1992. This verified nurses as personally accountable for their own clinical decision-making and allowed for the development of nursing practice roles. The implication of this publication has been far-reaching in the speciality of gastrointestinal nursing, especially with the development of nurse consultants (NHSE 1999), clinical nurse specialists, nurse practitioners and nurse endoscopists over the last 10 years.

Nurses now commonly perform diagnostic tests and prescribe specific medications in gastroenterology which were previously the enclave of the medical fraternity (http://www.doh.gov.uk/supplementaryprescribing/ accessed 8 May 2004; NMC 2002a). Additionally, with an increased understanding of organic gastrointestinal conditions and the widespread recognition of the need for psychosocial support for gastrointestinal patients, in areas such as inflammatory bowel disease, advanced gastrointestinal nurse consultants, nurse specialists and nurse practitioners have evolved to deal with holistic patient care in these conditions.

The scope of gastrointestinal nursing

Gastrointestinal nursing is a distinct specialism within nursing in which nurses work alongside their medical and surgical colleagues in gastroenterology. Therefore gastroenterology nurses work with a wide range of patients from those suffering from minor and acute gastrointestinal disorders through chronic conditions to those requiring major surgery and treatment for malignant disease. Gastrointestinal nurses therefore support patients with distressing symptoms and those requiring endoscopic examination (nurses increasingly performing these themselves) and provide perioperative support.

At present the gastrointestinal nurse may work in a variety of locations ranging from hospital ward to endoscopy unit, outpatient setting and in the community. The role of specific nurses depends upon their basic nursing background, specialised formal education and clinical experiences.

The question as to what distinguishes a gastrointestinal nurse from other nurses requires attention. Gastrointestinal nursing can be defined as the nursing care of patients with established or suspected gastrointestinal conditions. The practice of gastrointestinal nursing requires application of the nursing process and includes nursing diagnosis. Several disciplines contribute to the basis of gastrointestinal nursing practice, including biological sciences, microbiology, behavioural sciences, communication skills and ethics. The work of Benner (1984) described the development of practice from novice to expert in nursing. The question arises of what constitutes expertise in gastrointestinal nursing. All gastrointestinal nurses will have had a grounding in the above-mentioned disciplines in the preregistration programmes and it is this platform that is built upon within the specialism of gastrointestinal nursing. One of the main differences between an experienced gastrointestinal nurse and a general nurse lies in their use of information when making judgements. Expertise develops as the gastrointestinal nurse practitioner begins to accumulate many similar instances of personal clinical experiences about particular care issues and formulates them into a body of experiential knowledge that is generalisable to other situations and the development of evidence-based practice.

Gastrointestinal nurses therefore assume responsibility for assessing, planning, implementing and evaluating nursing care for gastrointestinal patients, whether in the paediatric or adult setting. Generally, they are professionally autonomous in the clinical setting, documentation, teaching and research and care of equipment. These factors will have a direct effect upon the quality of nursing care provided. Additionally, responsibilities of the present-day gastrointestinal nurse may include those shown in Box 1.1.

Box 1.1   Responsibilities of the gastrointestinal nurse.

- Establishment of nursing assessment/diagnosis
- Health educator
- Nurse education
- Establishment of nursing priorities
- Ensure safe patient care
- Ethical decision maker
- Preparation for gastrointestinal procedures
- Undertake diagnostic investigations (oesophageal manometry)
- Perform diagnostic procedures (rigid sigmoidoscopy)
- Assist medical practitioners with investigations (insertion of PEG tubes)
- Monitor patients following procedures (post liver biopsy)
- Perform diagnostic tests (monitor stool samples for faecal occult blood)
- Member of patient support groups
- Collaborate with other health care professionals
- Prescription of specific medications
- Researcher

Box 1.2   Aspects of advanced gastrointestinal practice.

- Perform comprehensive physical assessments
- Order and perform diagnostic investigations (flexible sigmoidoscopy, endoscopy)
- Prescribe, administer and evaluate pharmacological treatment regimes
- Contribute to evidence-based (nursing) practice
- Establish medical and nursing diagnosis (nurse-led clinics)
- Multi-disciplinary collaboration (medics and professions allied to medicine)

Nursing practice will be influenced by the patient's emotional status and the needs of relatives and next of kin for support, assistance and information.

In advanced practice the gastrointestinal nurse may be required to carry out some of the aspects shown in Box 1.2.

The nurse practitioner in gastroenterology will develop a range of practice-based skills, which are built upon generic nursing skills.

Patient care in gastrointestinal nursing

The role of gastrointestinal nurses involves meeting the physical, psychosocial and emotional needs of their patients. As the gastrointestinal system comprises several organs with a range of functions, gastrointestinal disorders can produce a range of diverse symptoms, including those shown in Box 1.3.

Many of these symptoms cause considerable embarrassment and can lead to major disruption of the quality of life of patients. It is important to provide all patients with clear, understandable information and reassurance. Nursing assessment will provide vital information about specific fears and concerns of the patient prior to and during potentially unpleasant and often undignified investigations or treatments.

Box 1.3 Gastrointestinal symptoms.

- Abdominal pain
- Anorexia
- Weight loss
- Dysphagia
- Dyspepsia
- Vomiting
- Diarrhoea
- Constipation

Box 1.4 Pre-procedural documentation in gastroenterology.

Pre-procedural documentation includes:
- Presenting gastrointestinal complaint/symptoms
- Patient vital observations
- Physical assessment of patient
- Psychosocial assessment of the patient (i.e. levels of anxiety)
- Current medications
- Past medical history
- Risk factors (i.e. previous allergic reactions)/anaesthetic history
- Prophilactic medication (i.e. antibiotic pre-ERCP)
- Consent for treatment/investigation

If a patient requires sedation during a procedure, such as endoscopy, the gastrointestinal nurse should be on hand to assess the patient's response to the sedation and the procedure and intervene where necessary. Patient monitoring continues for the nurse after the procedure, as patients will often require time to recover from the possible effects of sedation or from the potential complications that may be related to treatment or investigation of gastrointestinal conditions. Another responsibility relates to the documentation of nursing practice via records, care plans and reports (NMC 2002b). Documentation requirements may vary from one hospital to the next according to specific institutional policies. For the purpose of this text documentation is examined for a gastrointestinal outpatient at three specific stages of the patient journey, pre-procedural, procedural and post-procedural. Pre-procedural documentation is summarised in Box 1.4, procedural documentation in Box 1.5 and several elements of post-procedural documentation in Box 1.6.

Box 1.5 Procedural documentation.

- Nature of procedure
- Staff involved in procedure
- Equipment used in procedure (i.e. endoscope log number)
- Medication and fluids administered during procedure
- Unusual events
- Vital observations throughout procedure
- Type of specimen/biopsy obtained
- Post-procedural assessment

Box 1.6   Post-procedural documentation.

- Physical condition
- Psychosocial status (emotional well-being)
- Wound status (if applicable)
- Level of consciousness (if sedation has been given)
- Post-procedural medication
- Post-procedural intravenous fluids
- Unusual events following procedure
- Discharge instructions for patients

Surgery in gastrointestinal nursing

Surgery on the gastrointestinal tract is always invasive to some degree and, while minimally invasive procedures are now more common, for instance for biliary surgery, surgery is never without its risks to the patient and is rarely performed without heightening anxiety in the patient. In both regards nurses have a major role to play. Nurses can reinforce the explanations of the need for surgery given by surgical staff; these may not have been fully understood by an anxious patient. In terms of gastrointestinal surgery, good post-operative care is required with particular attention to the possible development of peritonitis. Frequently patients leave surgery with both drains and intravenous infusions and good fluid balance is an important aspect of post-surgical care in addition to monitoring for signs of post-surgical shock and infection.

Surgery may not always have a positive outcome for the patient; there may be bad news in terms of malignancy and in surgery of both the small and large intestines there may be the possibility of a stoma. Whether the latter is expected or not, nurses – and often specialist nurses – have a major role to play in helping the patient to adapt to having a stoma, sometimes permanently. The patient with a stoma, in addition to psychosocial care, will require help with stoma hygiene and the fitting of ostomy bags in order that they may return to a relatively normal life. Where surgery has not had a positive outcome or there is the likelihood of further surgery, the nurse is well placed to offer support and explanations.

Educational preparation

It is important that nurses wishing to work within gastroenterology are familiar with the established educational prerequisite to work within this practice setting. Although these requirements vary throughout the UK, in general, nurses wishing to work in this speciality are required to possess an understanding of the following:

- normal anatomy and physiology of the gastrointestinal tract
- pathophysiology related to common gastrointestinal conditions
- pharmacology in gastrointestinal medicine
- behavioural sciences
- counselling skills and communication

Education and research in gastrointestinal nursing

Gastrointestinal nurses have a responsibility as educators. This educational role covers nursing students, trained and untrained nursing staff. The development of advanced nurse practitioners and specialists in gastrointestinal nursing has led to nurses being involved in medical education and the teaching of other professionals who are allied to medicine. Nurse specialists in inflammatory bowel disease who disseminate both their academic and clinical knowledge in presentations, papers and abstracts are a good example of this widening educational role of gastrointestinal nurses. Through presentation at professional meetings, such as the British Society of Gastroenterology or the Royal College of Nursing Gastroenterology and Stoma Care Nurses Forum, nurses meet the responsibility of expanding current knowledge. Related to education is research in gastrointestinal nursing. Nurses who embark upon research are required to have a sound knowledge of research techniques; this facilitates critical evaluation of published materials.

To achieve these responsibilities it is imperative for the gastrointestinal nurse to have a thorough understanding of normal gastrointestinal physiology and pathophysiology in common gastrointestinal conditions, and an understanding of the rationale behind investigation techniques and treatment regimes. This book will provide the gastrointestinal nurse with the appropriate information to assess, plan, implement and evaluate nursing care.

Gastrointestinal nursing: what this text adds

This introduction will help you to understand the purpose of this book and how to get the best out of it. It is written for a wide range of nurses: at one end of the spectrum for nurses who may have an interest in entering gastroenterology as a speciality, and at the other end for nurses working in the speciality who may wish to develop further into one of many roles such as nurse endoscopist, nurse practitioner or nurse consultant. These roles are developing in the UK at the time of writing and there has been a great demand for such a book to ensure at least a common level of knowledge in this area of work, for which many nurses will have had no special education or training.

From our experience as nurse educators we know that many nurses at pre-registration level, whether on diploma or degree programmes, struggle with the subjects of anatomy and physiology. There are many reasons for this, including the fact that nursing students may enter university with a very poor background in the life sciences. However, we also acknowledge our failings as teachers. In addition, there will be many nurses working in gastroenterology who have never been exposed to the appropriate level of teaching in the life sciences because they trained prior to the nursing educational reforms of the 1990s.

Structure, function and disorders of the gastrointestinal tract

For the above reasons, therefore, a significant proportion of this book is concerned with the structure and function of the gastrointestinal tract and the disorders which arise. The management of these disorders is described and, while we have tried to emphasise aspects of nursing where these are unique, our general approach has been to present medical, surgical and nursing management without differentiation. As already stated, with the possible exception of nurses who want to find out more about the speciality, this book is mainly directed at those in the speciality. Even those outside the speciality will be registered nurses and to list repeatedly aspects of nursing care which are generic to all patient groups would be unnecessary. This book is designed to fill gaps in the essential knowledge needed to nurse in this area; knowledge and experience of nursing generally is assumed. Furthermore, nurses work as part of a multidisciplinary team and to specify their part is unrealistic, particularly when the boundaries between nursing, medicine and surgery are being blurred by advanced nursing practice.

As far as possible, the chapters in Section 1 follow the pattern described in Figure 1.1.

Essential aspects of gastroenterology

After an overview of the gastrointestinal tract, each chapter takes one region of the tract and covers the anatomy and physiology, the range of disorders with causes and then describes the management of the disorder including medical, surgical and nursing care.

The chapters on the regions of the tract should all enable the reader to:

- Describe the region of the tract in anatomical terms
- Understand the physiological function of the region
- Identify the main disorders, and
- Relate the anatomy, physiology and disorders to nursing practice.

Section 2 covers essential aspects of gastroenterology and these include diagnostic tests, emergencies and pharmacology. Nurses are increasingly involved in the diagnostic aspects of gastroenterology, specifically nurse endoscopists

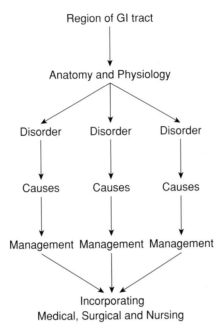

Figure 1.1 Schematic structure of the text.

and Chapter 10 considers endoscopy in some detail. Clearly, nurses are usually first on the scene in a gastrointestinal emergency. Some emergencies, such as haemorrhage, are common to several regions of the tract, therefore a range of emergencies is covered in Chapter 11. While specific drugs are mentioned throughout the book, the pharmacological aspects of gastroenterology are considered overall in Chapter 12. In addition to knowing which drugs are prescribed for which conditions and being able to list side-effects and interactions, nurses are increasingly required to understand how drugs work and to have a deeper knowledge of pharmacology, and this is commensurate with the development of nurse prescribers, especially in gastroenterology.

Living with gastrointestinal disorders

The final section of the book, Section 3, looks at living with gastrointestinal disorders. Chapter 13 covers the psychosocial aspects both as causes and consequences of gastrointestinal disorders, especially inflammatory bowel disease, and Chapter 14 looks at the impact of gastrointestinal disorders on quality of life. Clearly, there is a strong link between the two chapters. In common with developments in endoscopy and nurses prescribing, these are areas where nursing roles are extending with the development of nurse counsellors and the use of alternative treatments such as hypnotherapy.

Professional guidelines

Nurses are governed by a professional regulatory body called the Nursing and Midwifery Council (NMC), which was established in April 2002 and replaced the United Kingdom Central Council for Nursing, Midwifery and Health Visiting (UKCC). Wherever possible we refer readers to appropriate NMC documents. Where UKCC guidelines have not been superseded by NMC guidelines readers are referred to the relevant UKCC guidelines. The Appendix contains the latest version, at the time of publication, of the NMC Code of Professional Conduct reproduced with permission of the NMC.

FURTHER INFORMATION

This book is designed to be a stand-alone text. However, readers who wish to investigate specific aspects of structure and function or specific gastrointestinal disorders are referred to a range of standard texts, listed below. In addition, at the end of each chapter, specific references will be provided to relevant sections of these texts. To provide an evidence base for gastrointestinal nursing, appropriate sources such as websites, textbooks and journals are referred to in the text.

The following books were consulted in the preparation of this text:

Alexander, M., Fawcett, J.N. and Runciman, P. (2000) *Nursing Practice: Hospital and Home – the Adult.* Churchill Livingstone, Edinburgh.

Brooker, C. and Nicol, M. (2003) *Nursing Adults: the Practice of Caring.* Mosby, London.

Clancy, J. and McVicar, A.J. (1998) *Nursing Care: a Homeostatic Casebook.* Arnold, London.

Clancy, J. and McVicar, A.J. (2002) *Physiology and Anatomy: a Homeostatic Approach*, 2nd edition. Arnold, London.

Clancy, J., McVicar, A.J. and Baird, N. (2002) *Perioperative Practice: Fundamentals of Homeostasis.* Routledge, London.

Haslett, C., Chilvers, E.R., Boon, N.A. and Colledge, N.R. (2002) *Davidson's Principles and Practice of Medicine*, 19th edition. Churchill Livingstone, Edinburgh.

Higgins, C. (2000) *Understanding Laboratory Investigations: A Text for Nurses and Healthcare Professionals.* Blackwell Publishing, Oxford.

Hinchliff, S., Montague, S. and Watson, R. (1996) *Physiology for Nursing Practice*, 2nd edition. Baillière Tindall, London.

Kindlen, S. (2003) *Physiology for Health Care and Nursing.* Churchill Livingstone, Edinburgh.

Kumar, P. and Clark, M. (2002) *Clinical Medicine*, 4th edition. Saunders, Edinburgh.

McKenry, L.M. and Salerno, E. (1998) *Pharmacology for Nursing*, 20th edition. Mosby, St Louis.

Watson, R. (1999) *Essential Science for Nursing Students: An Introductory Text.* Baillière Tindall, London.

Watson, R. (2000) *Anatomy and Physiology for Nurses*, 11th edition. Baillière Tindall, London.

CONCLUSION AND ACKNOWLEDGEMENTS

We are responding to a demand for a book such as this and take full responsibility for any deficiencies. The book would not have been written without the support of Dr Kelvin Palmer, Dr Helen J. Dallal, Miss Tonks Fawcett and Ms Rosemary Patterson, or without the patience and support of Beth Knight at Blackwell Publishing. Anonymous reviewers also played a significant role in shaping the book. Special thanks to Linda S. Smith for indexing and to Gillian Kidd for her artwork. We hope this book is found useful by a wide range of nurses in gastroenterology and we will also be very glad to receive any feedback for future editions.

REFERENCES

Benner, P. (1984) *From Novice to Expert: Excellence and Power in Clinical Nuring Practice.* Addison-Wesley, Massachusetts.
NHSE (National Health Service Executive) (1999) *Nurse, Midwifery and Health Visitor Consultants*, HSC 1999/217 Department of Health, London.
NMC (2002a) *Guidelines for the Administration of Medicines.* Nursing and Midwifery Council, London.
NMC (2002b) *Guidelines for Records and Record Keeping.* Nursing and Midwifery Council, London.

Section 1
Structure, Function and Disorders of the Gastrointestinal Tract

Chapter 2
An Overview of the Gastrointestinal Tract

Chapter objectives

After reading this chapter you should be able to:

- Describe the general features of the gastrointestinal tract.
- Understand the range of functions of the gastrointestinal tract.

Introduction

The adult gastrointestinal tract consists of a continuous fibromuscular tube that extends from the mouth to the anus. The tract is in contact with the external environment at both ends.

The gastrointestinal system consists of the digestive tract (mouth, oesophagus, stomach and intestines) in association with the accessory digestive glands (salivary glands, pancreas and biliary system). The overall function of the digestive system is to transfer the nutrients in food from the external environment to the internal environment. Once in the body, the nutrients can be distributed to the cells of the body via the circulation. The waste material of digestion is also excreted via the circulation. Nutrients, water and salts are absorbed from digested food and all products that cannot be absorbed are retained in the digestive tract until they are eliminated. The gastrointestinal tract is regulated by both the autonomic nervous system and hormonal mechanisms, which act in conjunction with a variety of gastrointestinal peptides (hormones, neurocrines or paracrines).

In this chapter the general principles and the basic mechanisms involved in the overall function of the digestive system will be examined. Figure 2.1 illustrates both the component organs of the gastrointestinal tract and the accessory organs that are required for the digestive system to function.

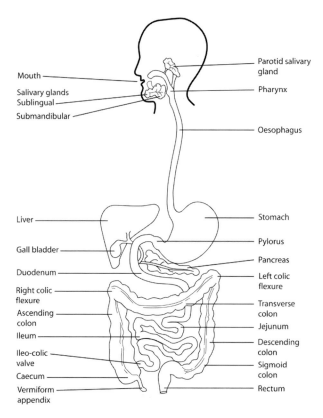

Figure 2.1   Component organs and accessory organs of the gastrointestinal tract. Reproduced with permission from Watson (2000).

Box 2.1   Generalised layers of the gastrointestinal tract.

- mucosa
- submucosa
- muscularis
- serosa (fibrous outer layer)

Structure of the gastrointestinal tract

The digestive tract wall consists of four structural layers (see Box 2.1). These four layers are present in all areas of the tract from the oesophagus to the anus, with some functional adaptations throughout (Figure 2.2).

The mucosa is the innermost layer, that is, the layer nearest to the lumen of the tube, and it exhibits a great deal of variation throughout the tract. Mucus stratified epithelial cells line the lumen (except in the oesophagus), and it is from this layer that all glands develop. Mucus secreting cells are situated throughout the epithelium. These cells are subjected to a tremendous amount of frictional wear and tear. The epithelial cells lie on a sheet of connective

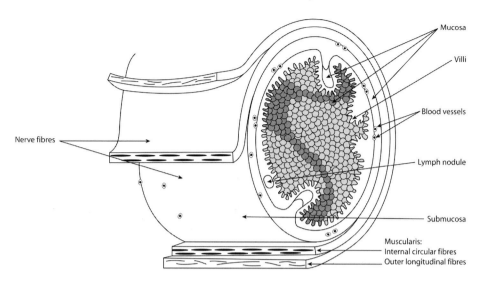

Figure 2.2   Four structural layers of digestive tract wall. Reproduced with permission from Hinchliff *et al.* (1996).

tissue called the lamina propria. Distal to this there is a thin layer of muscle tissue called the muscularis mucosa. Throughout the mucosa are patches of lymphoid tissue, which provide a defensive function.

The submucosa lies distal to the mucosa and consists of loose connective tissue, which supports blood vessels, lymphatics and nerve fibres.

The muscularis layer, as its name suggests, is formed of muscle fibres. The muscle fibres in the gastrointestinal tract are referred to as smooth, involuntary, unstriated or visceral muscle fibres.

The serosa is the outermost, protective layer, formed of connective and squamous tissue. The serosa contains blood vessels, neurones and lymphatics.

Blood supply

An adequate supply of blood to the digestive system is essential to serve the normal metabolic functions and also to provide a route for nutrients to get from the digestive tract to the systemic circulation. The arteries supplying the abdominal organs of the digestive system are the coeliac and superior and inferior mesenteric arteries. The coeliac artery branches to give rise to the gastric, splenic and hepatic arteries that provide blood to the stomach, pancreas, spleen and liver. The mesenteric arteries supply the intestines.

The branches of the main arteries, which supply the gastrointestinal tract, give rise to smaller branches, which penetrate the organs. These smaller branches divide to give rise to an extensive network of arterioles in the submucosa. These in turn lead to mucosal arterioles, which supply blood to the capillaries.

Venous blood from the stomach, pancreas, spleen and liver is collected together and routed through the liver via the hepatic portal vein. Blood from the remainder of the digestive tract (oesophagus and rectum) escapes the hepatic filter and drains directly into the venous system.

PHYSIOLOGY OF THE DIGESTIVE SYSTEM

The unique physiological processes that take place in the digestive system are digestion, absorption, secretion, motility and excretion.

Digestion is the process whereby large food molecules are broken down to smaller ones. Food is ingested as large pieces of matter containing substances such as protein and starch which are unable to cross the cell membranes of the gut epithelium. Before these complex molecules can be utilised they are degraded to smaller molecules, such as glucose and amino acids, which can be absorbed from the gastrointestinal system into the bloodstream.

The mixture of ingested material and secretions in the gastrointestinal tract contains water, minerals and vitamins as well as fats, carbohydrates and proteins. The products of digestion, other small dissolved molecules, ions and water are transported across the epithelial cell membranes, mainly in the small intestine. This is the process of absorption. The transported molecules enter the blood or lymph for circulation to the tissues. This process is central to the digestive system, and the other physiological processes of the gastrointestinal tract, such as elimination, subserve it.

Food which is ingested travels along the gastrointestinal tract to the appropriate sites for mixing, digestion and absorption to occur. Most of the gastrointestinal tract is lined by two layers of smooth muscle; contraction of this muscle mixes the contents of the lumen and moves them through the tract. Motility in the digestive system is under neural and hormonal control.

Exocrine glands secrete enzymes, ions, water, mucins and other substances into the digestive tract. The glands are situated within the gastrointestinal tract, in the walls of the stomach, small intestine and large intestine, or outside it in the case of salivary glands, pancreas and liver. Secretion in all regions of the gastrointestinal tract is controlled by nerves and hormones.

Peptides of the gastrointestinal tract

Some of the functions of the gastrointestinal tract are regulated by peptides, derivatives of amino acids and a variety of mediators released from nerves. These functions include contraction and relaxation of the smooth muscle wall and the sphincters (physiological 'gatekeepers' of the gastrointestinal tract); secretion of enzymes for digestion; secretion of fluids and electrolytes; and growth of the tissues of the gastrointestinal tract.

All gastrointestinal hormones are peptides, i.e. small molecules comprising up to 50 amino acids. It is important, however, to realise that not all peptides found in the digestive tract are hormones. The gastrointestinal peptides can be divided into hormones, paracrines and neurocrines, depending on the method by which the peptide is delivered to its target site.

Hormones are peptides released from endocrine cells of the gastrointestinal tract. They are secreted into the portal circulation, pass through the liver and enter the systemic circulation. The systemic circulation then delivers the hormone to target cells with receptors for that specific hormone. These target cells may be in the gastrointestinal tract itself (e.g. gastrin acts upon the parietal cells of the stomach to stimulate acid secretion), or the target cells may be located in another region of the body (e.g. gastric inhibitory peptide acts upon the β cells of the pancreas to cause insulin secretion). Several criteria must be met for a substance to qualify as a gastrointestinal hormone:

- The substance must be secreted in response to a physiological stimulus and carried in the bloodstream to a distant site, where it produces a physiological action.
- The hormone's action must be independent of any neural activity.
- The hormone must have been isolated, purified and chemically identified.

Four gastrointestinal peptides are classified as hormones: gastrin, cholecystokinin (CCK), secretin and gastric inhibitory peptide (GIP). These are discussed in more detail in Chapters 4 and 8.

Most paracrines, with the exception of histamine, are peptides secreted by endocrine cells of the gastrointestinal tract. In contrast to hormones, however, the paracrines act locally within the same tissue that secretes them. Paracrine substances reach their target cells by diffusing short distances through interstitial tissue, or they are carried short distances in capillaries. The only gastrointestinal peptide with a known paracrine function is somatostatin, which has an inhibitory effect throughout the gastrointestinal tract in that it reduces motility and secretion of digestive juices.

Neurocrines are synthesised in neurones of the gastrointestinal tract and are released in response to an action potential. Following release, the neurocrine diffuses across the synapse and acts upon its target cell. There are many neurocrines in the gastrointestinal tract including acetylcholine, noradrenalin and vasoactive intestinal peptide (VIP). The sources and actions of these neurocrines are summarised in Table 2.1.

Innervation of the gastrointestinal tract

The gastrointestinal tract is also regulated by the autonomic nervous system, which has an intrinsic component and an extrinsic component. The extrinsic component is the sympathetic and parasympathetic innervation of the gastrointestinal tract. The intrinsic component is called the enteric nervous system. The enteric system is wholly contained within the wall of the gastrointestinal tract in the submucosal and myenteric plexuses.

Table 2.1 Neurocrines of the enteric nervous system.

Neurocrine	Source	Action
Acetylcholine	Cholinergic neurons	Contraction of smooth muscle Relaxation of sphincters ↑ Salivary secretion ↑ Gastric secretion ↑ Pancreatic secretion
Noradrenalin	Adrenergic neurons	Relaxation of smooth wall Contraction of sphincters ↑ Salivary secretion
Vasoactive intestinal peptide (VIP)	Neurons of mucosa	Relaxation of smooth muscle ↑ Intestinal secretion ↑ Pancreatic secretion

↑ = increase in production of secretion.

Parasympathetic innervation

Parasympathetic nervous innervation is supplied by both the vagus nerve and the pelvic nerve. The pattern of parasympathetic innervation is consistent with its function. The vagus nerve innervates the upper portions of the gastrointestinal tract (upper third of oesophagus, wall of stomach, small intestine and ascending colon), whilst the pelvic nerve innervates the lower portions of the system (striated muscle of external anal canal and walls of the transverse, descending and sigmoid colons).

Postganglionic neurons of the parasympathetic nervous system are classified as either cholinergic or peptidergic. Cholinergic neurons release acetylcholine as the main neurotransmitter and peptidergic neurons release one of several peptides, including VIP.

Sympathetic innervation

Preganglionic cholinergic fibres of the sympathetic nervous system synapse in ganglia outside the gastrointestinal tract. Four sympathetic ganglia serve the gastrointestinal tract: coeliac, superior mesenteric, inferior mesenteric and hypogastric. Postganglionic fibres, which are adrenergic, leave the sympathetic ganglia and synapse on ganglia in the myenteric and submucosal plexus, or they directly innervate smooth muscle, endocrine or secretory cells.

Intrinsic innervation

The intrinsic or enteric nervous system can direct all functions of the gastrointestinal tract, even in the absence of extrinsic innervation. The enteric nervous system is located in the myenteric and submucosal plexus and controls the secretory, contractile and endocrine functions of the gastrointestinal tract.

Motility (movement) in the gastrointestinal tract

Motility refers to contraction and relaxation of the walls and sphincters of the gastrointestinal tract. Motility involves the grinding and mixing of ingested food in preparation for digestion and absorption; it then propels the food along the gastrointestinal tract. Smooth muscle in the gastrointestinal tract enables:

- Contractile tone to be maintained even in the absence of food.
- Activity to be increased and decreased as necessary.
- The tract to distend to accommodate different volumes.

The control of motility and secretion of smooth muscle in the gastrointestinal tract is by neural, hormonal and paracrine mechanisms. The neural control is via the extrinsic nerves of the autonomic nervous system. In most instances the mediators of neural or hormonal control are peptides.

Skeletal muscle which is present in the pharynx, upper section of the oesophagus and the external anal sphincter is under voluntary control and is involved in the initiation of swallowing and the final stage of defaecation.

Digestion and absorption

Digestion and absorption are the ultimate functions of the gastrointestinal tract. Digestion is the chemical breakdown of ingested foods into absorbable molecules. The digestive enzymes are secreted in salivary, gastric, and pancreatic juices as well as the mucosa of the small intestine.

Absorption is the movement of nutrients, water and electrolytes from the lumen of the intestine into the blood system. There are two distinct paths for absorption, a cellular path and a paracellular path. In the cellular path, the substance must cross the gastrointestinal luminal membrane, enter the intestinal epithelial cell, and then be extruded from the cell into the blood. Paracellular absorption involves the movement of substances across the tight junctions between the intestinal epithelial cells, through the lateral intercellular spaces, and then into the blood.

The structure of the intestinal mucosa is ideally suited for absorption of large quantities of nutrients. Structural features called villi and microvilli increase the surface area of the small intestine, maximising the exposure of nutrients to digestive enzymes and to the absorptive surface.

The epithelial cells of the small intestine have the highest turnover rate of any cells in the body. They are replaced every 3–6 days.

Constituents of food

The body needs food to provide energy. Vitamins and minerals are necessary to maintain good health. The main food groups are carbohydrate, fat and protein. In addition, water is essential to replace fluid, which is continually being lost by the body. There are in total six essential foodstuffs with which the body must be constantly supplied, each of which are examined here in turn.

Essential foodstuffs are:

- protein
- carbohydrate
- fat
- water
- mineral salts
- vitamins

These foodstuffs must be digested and absorbed. Food must therefore be of such a nature that it can be digested, i.e. broken down by digestive juices into substances that can pass into the bloodstream, and be carried to various tissues for their use.

Carbohydrates

The foods required for energy and heat within the body are called carbohydrate foods because they contain carbon, hydrogen and oxygen. Carbohydrates include sugar and starch and they are the chief source of body fuel.

Fats

Fatty foods provide energy and heat, which serve as body fuel. Fats also provide food stores, the adipose tissue of the body and protective coverings for some organs. It is recommended that dietary fat should account for less than 35% of total energy intake.

Proteins

Proteins are the most complicated foodstuffs, containing nitrogen in addition to hydrogen, carbon, oxygen and in some cases sulphur and phosphorus. They are called nitrogenous foodstuffs as they are the only ones which contain the element nitrogen. Protein is necessary in the diet to build and replace the protoplasm of body cells. Proteins are composed of polypeptides, derived from amino acids. There are 20 amino acids, although each protein contains only some of these. Humans require approximately 0.75 g of protein per kg of body weight per day.

Water

Water is essential for life as it forms nearly two-thirds of the human body and is present in most of the foods we eat. The average amount of water in the human body is about 45 litres (30 litres inside the cells – intracellular – and 15 litres outside the cells – extracellular – i.e. tissue fluid in the plasma). The main functions of water in the body are:

- excretion of waste products
- making digestive and lubricating fluids
- building of body tissues and body fluids
- temperature control (i.e. evaporation of sweat)

If the body is depleted of fluid the signs and symptoms of dehydration may appear; these include:

- thirst
- dry mouth
- slack elastic skin
- sunken eyes
- low blood pressure

The body requires 2–3 litres of water every day and the amount of fluid taken into the body must be balanced by the output.

Mineral salts

Mineral salts are essential for normal metabolism. Salts are produced by the action of an acid on a mineral.

An electrolyte is a dissolved salt (a mineral salt), which is capable of conducting electricity. The two major electrolytes are sodium (Na^+) and potassium (K^+). The concentration of Na^+ is high in extracellular sites and low within cells (intracellular). In contrast K^+ is low in tissue fluids and high within cells. A correct balance of electrolytes is essential for normal function of body tissues and fluids.

Sodium is present in all tissues; it exists as sodium chloride in a concentration of nine grams per litre (0.9%) in all extracellular fluids. Sodium is derived from our food, particularly animal foodstuffs, and from the rock salt used in cooking.

Potassium is present in all tissue cells, where it replaces the sodium of blood and tissue fluids and the source of the positively charged ions. Potassium is obtained from food, particularly plant foodstuffs.

Calcium is present in all tissues, particularly in bone, teeth and blood, and is necessary for the functioning of nerves and for muscle tone. It is obtained chiefly from milk, cheese, eggs and green vegetables. Adults require 400–500 mg daily.

Iron is essential for the formation of the haemoglobin in red blood cells. It is obtained from green vegetables, particularly spinach and cabbage, egg yolk and red meats. Men require 10 mg daily; women require more, 10–15 mg daily, because of menstrual blood loss.

Iodine is required for the formation of thyroxin by the thyroid gland. It is obtained from seafood and is also present in green vegetables.

Calcium, iron and iodine are the only minerals which may be insufficient in the diet.

Vitamins

Vitamins are also essential to normal health because they are necessary for a range of metabolic functions; they are of no value to the body as a fuel or as building material. Vitamins are present in small quantities in living foodstuff and are only required in minute traces each day. Vitamins are classified as fat soluble and water soluble; vitamins A, D, E and K are fat soluble, the other vitamins including B and C are soluble in water.

Vitamin A is present in all fatty foods, e.g. milk, cheese and fish liver oils. It can be made in the body from a substance called carotene, which is present in carrots and tomatoes. Vitamin A is needed for normal function of the retina and to fight infection. Correspondingly a lack of vitamin A causes visual loss, stunted growth and a lowered resistance to infection.

Vitamin D is found in dairy produce and also in fatty fish such as herring. Cod liver oil and halibut liver oil are very rich in vitamin D. Vitamin D can also be built up in the body; the ultraviolet rays from the sun act on a fatty substance in the skin called ergosterol, which produces vitamin D. Vitamin D is necessary, with calcium, for the formation of bone. Lack of vitamin D and/or calcium leads to rickets in childhood, osteomalacia and osteoporosis in adults.

Vitamin E is present in vegetable oils and is found in egg yolk and milk. Vitamin E is necessary for normal functions of the nervous system, reproduction and muscle development.

Vitamin K is fat soluble and can be obtained from green vegetables and liver. It is required for the production of blood clotting factors in the liver. Vitamin K is synthesised in the intestine by colonic bacterial action.

Vitamin B is a complex of several closely related compounds. These are found particularly in the husks and germs of cereals and pulses, in yeast and yeast extracts and to a lesser extent in vegetables, fruit, milk, eggs and meat. The chief factors in the vitamin B complex are:

- Vitamin B_1 (thiamine) is essential for carbohydrate metabolism and controls the nutrition of nerve cells.
- Vitamin B_2 (riboflavin) is essential for the proper functioning of cell enzymes.
- Vitamin B_6 (pyridoxine) is necessary for protein metabolism.
- Vitamin B_{12} (cyanocobalamin) is the anti-anaemic substance or factor absorbed by the villi of the small intestine and stored in the liver. It is satisfactorily absorbed only in the presence of intrinsic factor produced by the cells in the lining of the stomach. Vitamin B_{12} is essential for the proper development of red cells in the red bone marrow and of nervous tissue.

Folic acid is required in the body for the maturation of red blood cells. It is derived from green vegetables.

Vitamin C (ascorbic acid) is water soluble and is found in citrus fruits (oranges, grapefruits and lemons), green vegetables and potatoes. Vitamin C is important in tissue respiratory activity, wound repair and resistance to infection, and it affects the condition of capillary walls. Lack of vitamin C causes scurvy, a condition which used to be common in sailors on long sea voyages. Scurvy is occasionally seen today in older people who have not been feeding themselves properly.

Roughage is an indigestible part of food. It remains in the bowel and stimulates it to empty itself. Roughage is the fibrous part of food, giving it bulk and stimulating bowel action, thus preventing constipation.

Conclusion

From this general overview of the gastrointestinal tract it can be seen that it is important to several crucial functions in the body and ones with which we are very familiar: eating, drinking and elimination. The two main activites of the gastrointestinal tract – motility and absorption, both necessary for the digestive functions of the tract – are generally insensible. However, pathological conditions of the gastrointestinal tract affect these activities, leading to disorders in the functions of the tract with attendant discomfort, poor nutrition, embarrassment and distress. The nursing role, in addition to supporting the medical and surgical interventions related to the gastrointestinal tract, is to support patients through the consequences of disorders of the tract and for this to be possible, at least a working knowledge of the anatomy, physiology and disorders of the tract is required. The following chapters take you through the tract from the oesophagus to the rectum and include the ancillary organs of digestion (liver, pancreas and gall bladder).

BACKGROUND READING

Additional reading to support the material in this chapter can be found in the relevant sections of the following texts:

Clancy, J. and McVicar, A.J. (2002) *Physiology and Anatomy: a Homeostatic Approach*, 2nd edition. Arnold, London (Chapter 10).

Hinchliff, S., Montague, S. and Watson, R. (1996) *Physiology for Nursing Practice*, 2nd edition. Baillière Tindall, London (Chapter 5.1).

Kindlen, S. (2003) *Physiology for Health Care and Nursing*. Churchill Livingstone, Edinburgh (Chapter 9).

Watson, R. (1999) *Essential Science for Nursing Students: An Introductory Text*. Baillière Tindall, London (Chapter 2).

Watson, R. (2000) *Anatomy and Physiology for Nurses*, 11th edition. Baillière Tindall, London (Section V).

Chapter 3
The Oesophagus

Chapter objectives

After reading this chapter you should be able to:

- Describe the anatomy and physiology of the oesophagus, including the lower and upper oesophageal sphincters.
- Understand motility in the oesophagus.
- Identify the range of clinical conditions associated with the oesophagus.
- Relate the corresponding pathophysiology, diagnosis and treatment for disorders of the oesophagus to nursing practice.

ANATOMY AND PHYSIOLOGY

The oesophagus is a thin-walled, muscular tube, approximately 25 cm in length and 2–3 cm in diameter in adults. An endoscopic view of a normal oesophagus is shown in Plate 1 (see colour plate section).

Control of swallowing (deglutition)

Swallowing can be divided into three phases:

- voluntary
- pharyngeal
- oesophageal

Voluntary phase
The tongue moves food backwards and upwards into the back of the mouth. This is initiated voluntarily but once it has been initiated it cannot be stopped voluntarily, it is a classical 'all or none' reflex.

Pharyngeal phase
As the food moves into the pharynx, it activates pressure receptors in the pharynx. These receptors send impulses via the trigeminal and glossopharyn-

geal nerves to the brain stem swallowing centre. Each impulse serves as a trigger for the swallowing reflex. This causes the elevation of the soft palate, which seals the nasal cavity and prevents food entering it. The swallowing centre inhibits respiration by raising the larynx and closing the glottis to prevent food entering the trachea. The upper oesophageal sphincter, which is closed at rest, opens during swallowing to allow the bolus of food to pass into the oesophagus. Immediately after the bolus has passed, the sphincter closes again, resealing the junction. The pharyngeal phase of swallowing lasts approximately one second (Figure 3.1).

Oesophageal phase

As the peristaltic waves commence in the oesophagus, the muscle of the lower oesophageal sphincter relaxes, opening the sphincter and allowing the food bolus to enter the stomach. The lower oesophageal sphincter muscle then contracts to reseal the junction. The lower oesophageal sphincter remains closed in the absence of peristalsis, preventing the reflux of the acidic contents of the stomach into the oesophagus (Figure 3.2).

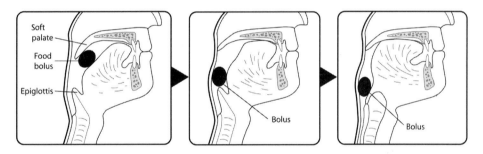

Figure 3.1   Pharyngeal phase of swallowing. Reproduced by permission of Hodder Arnold from Clancy and McVicar (2002).

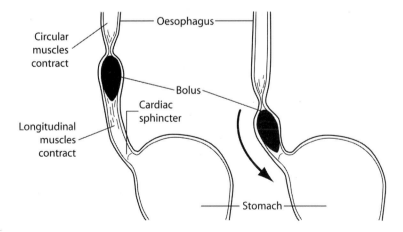

Figure 3.2   Oesophageal phase of swallowing. Reproduced by permission of Hodder Arnold from Clancy and McVicar (2002).

Anatomical arrangement of the oesophagus

The structure of the oesophagus is made up of three layers: the mucosa, submucosa and the muscularis. Unlike the bulk of the gastrointestinal tract, the oesophagus is not surrounded by serosa.

The innermost mucosal layer is composed of stratified squamous epithelium. Beneath the epithelium is the lamina propria, which is composed of connective tissue. At the upper and lower ends of the oesophagus the mucosa contains mucus-producing glands. A thin band of smooth muscle, the muscularis mucosa, separates the lamina propria from the underlying mucosa. The submucosa is the middle layer of the oesophagus and contains loose connective tissue with both elastic and fibrous components, as well as blood vessels and nerve fibres.

The arrangement of the muscularis layer in the oesophagus is similar to that of the rest of the digestive tract in that there is an inner circular layer and an outer longitudinal layer. Between the two muscular layers lies the intermuscular Auerbech's nerve plexus. However, only the lower two-thirds of the oesophagus is surrounded by smooth muscle. The upper third is surrounded by skeletal muscle.

The muscle tissue in the middle of the oesophagus is a transition zone of both skeletal and smooth muscles and this area covers as much as 35–45% of the length of the oesophagus.

At the upper end of the oesophagus is the upper oesophageal sphincter (hypopharyngeal sphincter). It is composed of skeletal cricopharyngeal muscle, which is a thickening of the circular muscular layer. At the lower end of the oesophagus, at the junction between the oesophagus and the stomach, is the lower oesophageal sphincter (gastro-oesophageal sphincter or cardiac sphincter); it comprises the distal 2–3 cm of the oesophagus. The lower oesophageal sphincter controls the passage of ingested food to the stomach.

Blood supply to the oesophagus

The oesophagus receives arterial blood via the oesophageal arteries of the aorta, the inferior thyroid artery and the left gastric artery. Blood is returned to the venous system by way of the left gastric, thyroid and azygous veins.

Neural control of the oesophagus

The oesophagus receives both sympathetic and parasympathetic innervation. The swallowing centre in the medulla oblongata initiates peristaltic contractions via the vagus (Xth crainial) nerve, which innervates the skeletal muscles in the upper oesophagus. The smooth muscle is innervated indirectly by neurons in the vagus nerve, which synapse with neurons in the myenteric plexus. The lower part of the oesophagus is believed to receive both sympathetic and parasympathetic innervation.

Motility in the oesophagus

When food is not being ingested, both oesophageal sphincters remain closed. The presence of a bolus of food in the pharynx opens the upper oesophageal sphincter and allows the food to pass into the oesophagus. A peristaltic wave consists of a wave of contraction of the circular muscle, followed by a wave of relaxation. These waves of contraction pass along the walls of the oesophagus and move foodstuff towards the stomach. Each peristaltic wave takes about nine seconds to travel the length of the oesophagus. Therefore it is not primarily gravity, but peristalsis, that moves food towards the stomach, although gravity does assist the process. Secondary peristalsis, which arises from within the oesophagus, is controlled by sympathetic stimulation.

DISEASES OF THE OESOPHAGUS

Pathophysiology of the oesophagus arises due to disorders of the skeletal muscle or the smooth muscle. Important disorders of the oesophagus include gastro-oesophageal reflux disease (GORD), motility disorders and gastric cancer.

Gastro-oesophageal reflux disease

Gastro-oesophageal reflux disease (GORD) is the most common cause of indigestion, affecting up to 30% of the general population. GORD develops when gastric or duodenal contents flow back into the oesophagus. Oesophageal reflux is only considered a pathological condition when it causes undesirable symptoms.

Clinical features of GORD

The most common symptoms of oesophageal reflux are dyspepsia, heartburn and regurgitation, which can be provoked by bending, straining or lying down. Waterbrash, which is salivation due to reflex salivary gland stimulation as acid enters the gullet, is often present. A history of weight gain is common. Some patients are woken at night by choking as refluxed fluid irritates the larynx. Other less common symptoms include dysphagia (difficulty swallowing), odynophagia (pain on swallowing), and symptoms of anaemia. A small number of patients present with atypical chest pain, which may be severe, can mimic angina and is probably due to reflux-induced oesophageal spasm.

Pathophysiology of GORD

Occasional episodes of GORD are common in health, particularly after eating. Gastro-oesophageal reflux disease develops when the oesophageal mucosa is exposed to gastric contents for prolonged periods of time, resulting in symptoms and, in a small proportion of cases, this leads to oesophagitis.

Abnormalities of the lower oesophageal sphincter related to GORD
In health the lower oesophageal sphincter is tonically contracted, relaxing only during swallowing. Some patients with GORD have reduced lower oesophageal sphincter tone, permitting reflux when intra-abdominal pressure rises. In others basal sphincter tone is normal but reflux occurs in response to frequent episodes of inappropriate sphincter relaxation.

Hiatus hernia
A hiatal hernia occurs when part of the stomach protrudes through the diaphragm and into the thoracic cavity. Such hernias are extremely common in older people and more common in women than in men. A hiatus hernia causes reflux because the pressure gradient between the abdominal and thoracic cavities, which normally pinches the hiatus, is lost. In addition the oblique angle between the cardia and oesophagus disappears. Many patients who have large hiatus hernias develop reflux symptoms, but the relationship between the presence of a hernia and symptoms is poor. Hiatus hernias are very common in individuals who have no symptoms, and some symptomatic patients have only a very small or no hernia.

Important features of a hiatus hernia include:

- Occur in 30% of the population over the age of 50 years.
- Often asymptomatic.
- Heartburn and regurgitation can occur.
- Gastric volumes may complicate large hernias.

The role of gastric contents in GORD
Gastric acid is the most important oesophageal irritant and there is a close relationship between acid exposure time and symptoms. Alkaline reflux, due to bile reflux following gastric surgery, is of uncertain importance.

Increased intra-abdominal pressure
Pregnancy and obesity are established predisposing causes. Weight loss commonly improves symptoms and patients should be encouraged to avoid tight-fitting garments.

Dietary and environmental factors
Dietary fat, chocolate, alcohol and beverages such as tea and coffee relax the lower oesophageal sphincter and may provoke symptoms. There is little

evidence to incriminate smoking or non-steroidal anti-inflammatory drugs (NSAIDs) as causes of gastro-oesophageal reflux disease.

Delayed oesophageal clearance
Defective oesophageal peristaltic activity can be seen in patients who have GORD. Poor oesophageal clearance leads to increased exposure to acid from the stomach.

Complications of GORD

Oesophagitis
Reflux oesophagitis is a chronic inflammatory process mediated by gastric acid and pepsin from the stomach as well as bile from the duodenum, which can result in ulceration of the mucosa and secondary fibrosis in the muscular wall. A range of endoscopic findings, from mild redness to severe bleeding ulceration with stricture formation, is recognised. There is a poor correlation between symptoms and histological and endoscopic findings. A normal endoscopy and normal oesophageal histology are perfectly compatible with significant gastro-oesophageal reflux disease. Plate 2 shows an endoscopic view of mild oesophagitis.

Other causes of oesophagitis: infectious diseases
Viruses, bacteria, fungi and mycobacterium can all cause oesophageal infection. The most common of these are candida. Oesophageal candidiasis occurs in debilitated patients and those taking broad-spectrum antibiotics or cytotoxic drugs. It is a particular problem in AIDS patients, who are also susceptible to a spectrum of oesophageal infections. Oesophageal candidiasis rarely develops in patients who do not have an underlying disease such as diabetes, immune deficiency or malignancy. The main symptoms of oesophageal candidiasis are dysphagia and odynophagia. Severe infection of the gullet can destroy oesophageal innervation, causing abnormal motility.

Corrosives
Accidental or suicidal ingestion of highly alkaline or acidic substances may result in injury to the oesophagus. The most common symptom is odynophagia, but patients may also complain of dysphagia and chest pain. Ingestion of caustic compounds is followed by painful burns of the mouth and pharynx and by extensive erosive oesophagitis. At the time of presentation, management is conservative, based upon analgesia and nutritional support. Vomiting should be avoided and endoscopy should not be done at this stage because of the high risk of oesophageal perforation. Following the acute phase, a barium swallow and X-ray examination is performed to demonstrate the extent of stricture formation. Endoscopic dilation is usually necessary, although it is difficult and hazardous because strictures are often long, tortuous and easily perforated.

Barrett's oesophagus

Barrett's oesophagus is defined as epithelial metaplasia in which the normal squamous epithelium of the oesophagus is replaced by one or more of the following types of columnar epithelium: a specialised columnar epithelium, a junctional type of epithelium; and/or a gastric type of epithelium. Barrett's oesophagus is thought to be a consequence of chronic gastro-oesophageal reflux.

Diagnosis of Barrett's oesophagus is made by endoscopic visualisation of the oesophageal mucosa, supported by examination of tissue biopsies. Barrett's oesophagus is recognised endoscopically as confluent areas or fingers of pink, gastric-like mucosa extending from the cardia of the stomach into the oesophagus. The prevalence of adenocarcinoma in patients with Barrett's oesophagus is reported to be in the region of 30 to 50 times that of the general population (Clark *et al.* 2000). Consequently patients discovered to have Barrett's changes during endoscopy are considered for endoscopic surveillance programmes. Patients with moderate dysplasia should undergo repeated biopsies at 6 to 12-monthly intervals. Patients found to have severe dysplasia usually have associated cancer and are usually referred for oesophageal surgery.

Anaemia

Iron deficiency anaemia occurs as a consequence of chronic, insiduous blood loss and can result from longstanding oesophagitis.

Benign oesophageal stricture

An oesophageal stricture is an abnormal formation of fibrous tissue that is usually at the lower end of the oesophagus. Fibrous strictures develop as a consequence of longstanding oesophagitis. Most patients are older and have poor oesophageal peristaltic activity. Progressive dysphagia is the most common clinical feature. Diagnosis is made by endoscopy and biopsies of the stricture are taken to exclude malignancy. Treatment of strictures may involve the use of weighted bougies, pneumatic balloon dilators or graduated plastic Savary-Gillard dilators. An endoscopic balloon dilation of a benign oesophageal stricture is shown in Plate 3.

Subsequent treatment usually involves long-term therapy with a proton pump inhibitor drug (i.e. omeprazole or lansoprazole) which should be prescribed to reduce the risk of recurrent oesophagitis and stricture formation. The patient should be advised to chew food thoroughly and it is also important to ensure that dentition is adequate.

Investigations for GORD

Investigation is advisable if patients present in middle or late age, if symptoms are atypical or if a complication is suspected. Endoscopy is the investigation of choice. This is done to exclude other upper gastrointestinal diseases that can mimic gastro-oesophageal reflux, and to identify complications. A normal endoscopy in a patient with compatible symptoms should not preclude treatment for gastro-oesophageal reflux disease.

When, despite endoscopy, the diagnosis is unclear or if surgical intervention is under consideration, 24-hour pH monitoring is indicated (see Chapter 9). This involves tethering a slim catheter with a terminal radiotelemetry pH-sensitive probe above the gastro-oesophageal junction. The intraluminal pH is recorded whilst the patient undergoes normal activities, and episodes of pain are noted and related to pH. A pH of less than 4 for more than 4% of the study time is diagnostic of reflux disease.

Management of GORD

The first-line nursing of patients with GORD should relate to behaviour modification and nurses should encourage the following recommendations:

- weight loss
- avoidance of tight-fitting garments
- avoidance of dietary items which the patient finds worsens symptoms
- elevation of the bed-head in those who experience nocturnal symptoms
- avoidance of late meals
- cessation of smoking

Antacids, which are said to produce a protective mucosal 'raft' over the oeso-phageal mucosa, are taken with considerable symptomatic benefit by most patients. H_2 receptor antagonist drugs, which reduce gastric acid secretion, help symptoms without healing oesophagitis. They are well tolerated and the timing of medication and dosage should be tailored to individual need.

Proton pump inhibitors are the treatment of choice for severe symptoms and for complicated reflux disease. These drugs irreversibly inhibit the proton pump, reducing the transport of hydrogen (H^+) ions out of parietal cells. Symptoms almost invariably resolve and oesophagitis heals in the majority of patients. Recurrence of symptoms is almost inevitable when therapy is stopped, and some patients require lifelong treatment.

Patients who fail to respond to medical therapy, those who are unwilling to take long-term proton pump inhibitors and those whose major symptom is severe regurgitation are considered for anti-reflux surgery.

Evidence-based guidelines for the management of GORD have been published by the Scottish Intercollegiate Guidelines Network (SIGN) (2003) and the British Society of Gastroenterology (BSG) (2002).

Mallory-Weiss tear

A Mallory-Weiss tear is a mucosal tear at the gastro-oesophageal junction. It is associated with complications of GORD, prolonged forceful vomiting, alcohol abuse and trauma. Typically patients present with vomiting of bright red blood. The amount of blood lost is usually fairly small and these patients are generally treated conservatively, allowing the bleeding to stop spontaneously. Profuse bleeding may require to be controlled endoscopically using a coagulating heater probe.

Motility disorders

Oesophageal motility disorders can be classified as either primary or secondary if the oesophageal abnormalities are features of a more generalised condition. Primary oesophageal motility disorders include achalasia and oesophageal spasm.

Achalasia

Achalasia is a condition that involves chronic and progressive obstruction to the passage of contents through the lower oesophageal sphincter. It is characterised by defective peristalsis in the oesophagus combined with an elevated lower oesophageal sphincter pressure which fails to relax in response to the oesophageal swallowing wave.

Clinical features of achalasia
Patients with achalasia present with dysphagia to solids and liquids, sometimes associated with pain, regurgitation and weight loss. It is an unusual disease affecting 1 in 100 000 of Western populations (Dent 2000). It usually develops in middle or late adult life and the aetiology is unknown. Dysphagia develops slowly, and is initially intermittent. It is worse for solids and is eased by drinking liquids, standing and moving around after eating. Heartburn does not occur, since the closed oesophageal sphincter prevents gastro-oesophageal reflux. Some patients experience episodes of severe chest pain due to oesophageal spasm ('vigorous achalasia'), although this disappears as the body of the oesophagus loses peristaltic activity. Patients may worry that this pain is related to heart disease and gastrointestinal nurses should be in the position to provide reassurance and support in such situations.

Investigations for achalasia
A chest radiograph may be abnormal in late disease, with widening of the mediastinum from gross oesophageal dilation and features of aspiration pneumonia. A barium swallow will display narrowing of the lower oesophagus. In late disease the oesophageal body is dilated, with absence of peristalsis. Manometry is diagnostic and may demonstrate the failure of relaxation in the lower oesophagus. The nurse should provide the patient with clear information prior to this investigation to allay potential concerns.

Management of achalsia
Symptoms of achalasia may be minimised by eating slowly, chewing well, drinking fluids with meals, and sitting up whilst eating.

Endoscopic treatment
Forceful pneumatic dilation using an endoscopically positioned balloon disrupts the oesophageal sphincter and improves symptoms in 80% of patients. Some patients require more than one dilation but those requiring frequent dilation are best treated surgically. Endoscopically directed injection of botulinum toxin into the lower oesophageal sphincter induces clinical remission, but late relapse is common.

Surgical treatment
Surgical myotomy ('Heller's operation') is carried out by open operation or by a laparoscopic approach and is an extremely effective, although more invasive, option. Both pneumatic dilation and myotomy may be complicated by gastro-oesophageal reflux, and this can lead to severe oesophagitis because oesophageal clearance is so poor in these patients. For this reason Heller's myotomy is sometimes accompanied by an anti-reflux operation. Acid-suppressing drug therapy, using a proton pump inhibitor, is often necessary following surgical or endoscopic intervention for achalasia.

   Evidence-based guidelines for the management of achalasia have been published in the *American Journal of Gastroenterology* (1999).

Other oesophageal motility disorders

Diffuse oesophageal spasm
Diffuse oesophageal spasm is a motility disorder of unknown cause and pathophysiology. Diffuse oesophageal spasm usually presents in late middle age with episodic chest pain, which may mimic angina, but is sometimes accompanied by transient dysphagia. Some cases occur in response to gastro-oesophageal reflux. Treatment is based upon the use of proton pump inhibitors when gastro-oesophageal reflux is present. Results of drug therapy are often disappointing and the alternatives of pneumatic dilation and surgical myotomy are also poor.

Benign oesophageal stricture
An oesophageal stricture is an abnormal formation of fibrous tissue in the oesophagus. Progressive dysphagia is the most common clinical feature. To exclude malignancy as the cause of the stricture, endoscopic examination and multiple biopsies are required. A benign oesophageal stricture is usually the consequence of GORD and occurs most often in older patients who have poor oesophageal clearance.

Oesophageal varices
See Chapter 7, The Liver.

Tumours of the oesophagus

Carcinoma of the oesophagus affects approximately five per 100 000 of the population per annum (Clark *et al.* 2000). Two-thirds of oesophageal tumours are squamous carcinomas and the rest are adenocarcinomas.

A number of aetiological factors are known to be associated with oesophageal tumours. The most frequent of these relate to heavy alcohol intake and smoking; acid reflux associated with chronic oesophagitis is also postulated as a causative factor.

Squamous cancer

Squamous cancer can arise in any part of the oesophagus from the post-cricoid region to the cardia. Almost all tumours above the lower third of the oesophagus are squamous cancers.

Adenocarcinoma

This arises in the lower third of the oesophagus from Barrett's oesophagus or from the cardia of the stomach. The incidence of this tumour is increasing, possibly because of the high prevalence of gastro-oesophageal reflux and Barrett's oesophagus in Western populations.

Clinical features of oesophageal cancer

Most patients have a history of progressive, painless dysphagia for solid foods. Others present acutely because of food bolus obstruction. In late stages weight loss is often extreme; chest pain or hoarseness suggest mediastinal invasion. Fistulation between the oesophagus and the trachea or bronchial tree leads to coughing after swallowing, pneumonia and pleural effusion. Physical signs may be absent but even at initial presentation cachexia, cervical lymphadenopathy or other evidence of metastatic spread are common.

Investigations for oesophageal cancer

The investigation of choice is upper gastrointestinal endoscopy with cytology and biopsy. A barium swallow demonstrates the site and length of the stricture but adds little useful information.

Once a diagnosis has been achieved, investigations are carried out to stage the tumour and define operability. A chest radiograph and abdominal ultrasound may show obvious metastases.

Management of oesophageal cancer

Survival rates in oesophageal cancer are very poor (Clark *et al.* 2000); only 6% of patients with oesophageal cancer survive for five years following diagnosis.

In patients with disease with no metastatic spread outside the oesophagus the five-year survival rate rises to between 15 and 20%. For disease confined to the oesophagus, surgery should be considered in fit patients. Surgery alone cures only 5–10%, but a combination of preoperative radiotherapy, chemotherapy and radical surgery is associated with five-year survival of 30–50% in selected patients. Approximately 90% of the patients have extensive disease at presentation; in these, treatment is palliative and based upon relief of dysphagia and pain. Surgically performed palliative procedures include excision and reconstruction or bypass. Endoscopically directed tumour ablation using laser therapy or alcohol injection and insertion of stents are the major methods of improving swallowing. Palliative radiotherapy may induce shrinkage of both squamous cancers and adenocarcinomas but risks worsening stricture formation and exacerbating dysphagia.

Psychological care is important for patients who have an inoperable tumour or an oesophageal obstruction. Nursing staff will be involved in providing nutritional support and ensuring patients receive appropriate analgesia to optimise health-related quality of life.

Evidence-based guidelines for the management of oesophageal cancer have been published by Allum *et al.* (2002).

Benign tumours

The commonest benign tumour is stromal cell tumour (leiomyoma). This is usually asymptomatic but may cause bleeding or dysphagia.

Conclusion

The function of the oesophagus is simply to act as a channel for the end of the process of swallowing and the beginning of digestion in the stomach, and it participates in this process for only a few seconds. However, problems in the oesophagus can cause long-term misery and discomfort. The problems of the oesophagus are extrinsic and intrinsic to the oesophagus. The extrinsic problems such as GORD are the result of the acidic contents of the stomach coming into contact with the mucosa of the oesophagus, which if prolonged leads to complications such as inflammation and cytological changes. Oesophageal varices (see Chapter 7) also arise extrinsically as a result of increased pressure in the hepatic portal system, which is a consequence of liver failure. Intrinsic changes range from problems of motility to benign and malignant tumours. These conditions are especially distressing as they result in difficulty with swallowing, one of the most fundamental aspects of our existence associated with the ingestion of food. Malignancy of the oesophagus is especially worrying due to its poor prognosis.

The nurse has a range of responsibilities with regard to patients who have disorders of the oesophagus. These range from psychosocial support through the provision of simple and accurate explanations – augmenting those of the medical profession – to patients with any disorder of the oesophagus. However, the nurse can also be an invaluable source of advice on lifestyle changes that patients can make to alleviate mild symptoms. Oesophageal investigations involve endoscopy, often with the patient sedated but conscious, and the nurse has a crucial role in supporting such patients with the provision of information and accompanying the patient throughout the procedure. Nurses are also increasingly developing expertise as advanced and independent practitioners in this area of gastroenterology. Finally, in the case of life-threatening conditions such as oesophageal malignancy, the nurse's role extends beyond the usual support of the patient to those around the patient such as friends and family.

BACKGROUND READING

Additional reading to support the material in this chapter can be found in the relevant sections of the following texts:

Alexander, M., Fawcett, J.N. and Runciman, P. (2000) *Nursing Practice: Hospital and Home – the Adult.* Churchill Livingstone, Edinburgh (Chapter 4).
Brooker, C. and Nicol, M. (2003) *Nursing Adults: the Practice of Caring.* Mosby, London (Chapter 22).
Clancy, J. and McVicar, A.J. (2002) *Physiology and Anatomy: a Homeostatic Approach,* 2nd edition. Arnold, London (Chapter 10).
Clancy, J., McVicar, A.J. and Baird, N. (2002) *Perioperative Practice: Fundamentals of Homeostasis.* Routledge, London (Chapter 2).
Haslett, C., Chilvers, E.R., Boon, N.A. and Colledge, N.R. (2002) *Davidson's Principles and Practice of Medicine,* 19th edition. Churchill Livingstone, Edinburgh (Chapter 17).
Hinchliff, S., Montague, S. and Watson, R. (1996) *Physiology for Nursing Practice,* 2nd edition. Baillière Tindall, London (Chapter 5.1).
Kindlen, S. (2003) *Physiology for Health Care and Nursing.* Churchill Livingstone, Edinburgh (Chapter 9).
Kumar, P. and Clark, M. (2002) *Clinical Medicine,* 4th edition. Saunders, Edinburgh (Chapter 6).
McKenry, L.M. and Salerno, E. (1998) *Pharmacology for Nursing,* 20th edition. Mosby, St Louis (Unit 11).
Watson, R. (2000) *Anatomy and Physiology for Nurses,* 11th edition. Baillière Tindall, London (Chapter 20).

EVIDENCE-BASED GUIDELINES

Allum, W.H., Griffin, S.M., Watson, A. and Colin-Jones, D. (2002) Guidelines for the management of oesophageal and gastric cancer. *Gut,* **50**, Suppl V, v1–v23 (http://www.bsg.org.uk/pdf_word_docs/ogcancer.pdf accessed 8 May 2004).

American College of Gastroenterology (1999) Diagnosis and management of achalasia. *American Journal of Gastroenterology*, **94**, 3406–12 (http://www.guideline.gov/summary/summary.aspx?doc_id=2197 accessed 8 May 2004).

BSG (2002) *Dyspepsia Management Guidelines*. British Society of Gastroenterology, London (http://www.bsg.org.uk/clinical_prac/guidelines/dyspepsia.htm accessed 8 May 2004).

SIGN (2003) *Dyspepia: a National Clinical Guideline*. Scottish Intercollegiate Guidelines Network, Edinburgh (http://www.sign.ac.uk/pdf/sign68.pdf accessed 8 May 2004).

REFERENCES

Clark, M.L., Talbot, I.C., Thomas, H.J.W. and Williams, C.B. (2000) Tumours of the gastrointestinal tract. In: *Concise Oxford Textbook of Medicine* (Leadingham, J.G.G. and Worrell, D.A., eds), pp. 577–84. Oxford University Press, Oxford.

Dent, J. (2000) Diseases of the oesophagus. In: *Concise Oxford Textbook of Medicine* (Leadingham, J.G.G. and Worrell, D.A., eds), pp. 526–30. Oxford University Press, Oxford.

Chapter 4
The Stomach

Chapter objectives

After reading this chapter you should be able to:

- Describe the anatomy and physiology of the stomach.
- Understand the motor and secretory functions of the stomach.
- Identify the range of clinical conditions associated with the stomach.
- Relate the corresponding pathophysiology, diagnosis and treatment of selected conditions of the stomach to nursing practice.

ANATOMY AND PHYSIOLOGY

The stomach is a dilated segment of the digestive tract located between the oesophagus and the small intestine (see Figure 4.1). The physiological processes of the stomach involve a complex combination of exocrine secretions and smooth muscle contractions. The stomach serves as a reservoir for food and digestive secretions. It mixes and delivers chyme to the small intestine and originates the signals for hunger and satiety.

The stomach is divided into five regions:

- cardia
- fundus
- body
- antrum
- pylorus

The portion of the stomach that immediately adjoins the oesophagus is the cardia. The gastric fundus is the dome-shaped part of the stomach that extends to the left above the cardia. Below the fundus is the gastric body, which is located on the upper lateral border of the stomach.

Below the body and extending to the pylorus is the antrum. The upper lateral border of the stomach is called the lesser curvature, and the lower lateral border is called the greater curvature.

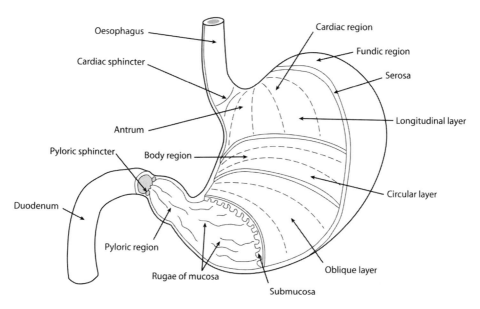

Figure 4.1 Anatomy of the stomach. Reproduced with permission of Hodder Arnold from Clancy and McVicar (2002).

The entry of food into the stomach is controlled by the lower oesophageal sphincter, or cardiac sphincter, which lies at the distal end of the oesophgaus and regulates the opening and closing of the oesophageal lumen.

At the distal end of the stomach is the pylorus. This has a thick, muscular wall that forms the pyloric sphincter, which controls the movement of stomach contents into the first part of the small intestine, the duodenum.

The gastric mucosa lines the interior of the stomach. Folds, known as rugae, are present on the inner surface of the stomach. The rugae allow the stomach to distend and hold a large quantity of foodstuff without any substantial increase in pressure. This allows the stomach to control the rate at which food enters the duodenum.

The structure of the stomach wall is similar to that throughout the rest of the digestive tract (see Chapter 2), except that the stomach has an oblique layer of muscle in addition to the circular and longitudinal layers in the muscularis mucosa. This additional layer facilitates distension of the stomach and storage of food. The external circular muscle layer is not evenly distributed throughout the stomach; it is relatively thin in the fundus and body regions and thicker in the antrum where strong muscular contractions aid the mechanical mixing of foods. The lining of the stomach is covered with a protective layer of columnar epithelial cells and these cells secrete mucus and alkaline fluid to protect the stomach from the acidic contents of the stomach.

Numerous gastric pits penetrate the surface of the stomach. These gastric pits are short ducts into which deep-lying gastric glands empty their secretions. These secretions enter the stomach via the neck of these ducts.

Secretory mucosa of the stomach

The mucosa of the stomach can be considered as two distinct regions: the upper region comprising the fundus and the body of the stomach, the oxyntic glandular region, and the lower antral and pre-pyloric region, which secretes the hormone gastrin. The secretory cells of the oxyntic region produce gastric juice. The major secretory cells present in this area are parietal (or oxyntic) cells, which secrete hydrochloric acid and intrinsic factor, which is a glycoprotein necessary for the absorption of vitamin B_{12}. The chief (or peptic) cells secrete pepsinogen, the precursor of the proteolytic enzyme pepsin.

The antrum and pylorus contain the pyloric glands; these glands contain mucous cells, which secrete mucus and pepsinogens, and G cells, which secrete gastrin. The pyloric and cardiac glands also have enterochromaffin cells, which secrete serotonin. The gastric mucosa also contains nine different types of endocrine cells, which secrete hormonal products such as glucagons and somatostatin. Both parietal and pyloric glands secrete bicarbonate.

Composition of gastric juice

The adult human secretes approximately two litres of gastric juice per day. Eating food stimulates the stomach to secrete gastric juice. Gastric juice is isotonic with blood plasma but the concentrations of its various constituents vary with the rate of flow: the higher the rate the more acid the juice. Following ingestion of a meal the chyme becomes more acidic; the acidity can reach pH 2.0. Maximum acid secretion can be induced by an injection of histamine; this procedure is used clinically to assess the secretory function of the stomach. Absence of hydrochloric acid secretion is known as achlorhydria and is seen when oxyntic cells have been damaged. This is usually associated with a lack of intrinsic factor, resulting in vitamin B_{12} deficiency and pernicious anaemia.

Motility

The movements of the stomach serve two basic functions: mixing and grinding of food, which takes place in the distal areas, and the controlled emptying of the gastric contents into the small intestine.

When a meal is ingested, weak peristaltic waves begin in the body of the stomach, pushing food into the antrum. Gradually these contractions become more intense, especially in the antral region. This contractile activity is responsible for the churning of food material and mixing with gastric juice. Thus, solid materials are progressively reduced to a semi-fluid material called chyme. Normally, peristalsis moves chyme slowly towards the pylorus at a rate of about three waves per minute.

Only a small proportion of chyme that is advanced towards the pylorus moves through the pyloric sphincter and into the duodenum. The rest is propelled backward, colliding with larger food particles still present in the antrum and body of the stomach. Particles have to be smaller than 1 mm in diameter to pass into the duodenum. About 6–10 ml of chyme are emptied into the duodenum each minute. The physiological function of this sphincter is to allow carefully regulated emptying of gastric contents, whilst preventing regurgitation of duodenal contents into the stomach. This is of vital importance as the lining of the stomach may be damaged by the presence of intestinal juices (including bile). Gastric emptying is controlled by neural impulses, by the composition of the chyme and by the presence of hormones secreted in the small intestine.

Absorption in the stomach

Very few substances are absorbed in the stomach and the stomach is virtually impermeable to water. Aspirin and alcohol are the main substances that can be absorbed. Alcohol is lipid soluble and aspirin becomes more lipid soluble in the acidic environment of the stomach.

Control of gastric secretion

There are three phases of stimulation: the cephalic, gastric and intestinal phases.

Cephalic phase
During the cephalic phase, gastric acid and pepsinogen secretion is activated by the thought, sight, smell and taste of food. It is mediated entirely by the vagus nerve; if vagal innervation of the stomach is ligated, the cephalic phase is abolished. This response to the sight or smell of food is a conditioned reflex, a learned response based on previous experiences of food.

Gastric phase
The gastric phase, as the name suggests, occurs when food is in the stomach and the presence of food stimulates the release of gastric juice. The control of secretion of gastric juice involves both intrinsic and extrinsic nerves, hormones such as gastrin and paracrine mediators such as histamine.

Intestinal phase
The intestinal phase occurs when food enters the duodenum and the secretion and motility is inhibited by hormonal and neural mechanisms.

Hormonal control of gastric secretion
Gastrin is secreted from G cells in the stomach and stimulates the secretion of gastric juice, generally preparing the gastrointestinal tract for the digestion and absorption of food.

Gastrin acts upon a variety of cell types that possess specific receptors (i.e. H_2 receptors). One such cell is the oxyntic (parietal) cell in the stomach. The secretion of gastric acid and intrinsic factor by the oxyntic (parietal) cells is normally regulated in parallel, such that the stimulation of gastric acid is accompanied by an increase of intrinsic factor. Gastrin stimulates acid secretion by two mechanisms: directly through the oxyntic (parietal) cells and indirectly through the stimulation of the enterochromaffin cell to release histamine, which acts upon H_2 receptors in the oxyntic (parietal) cells to produce more acid.

Neural control of gastric secretion
The stomach is controlled by the intrinsic nerves in the internal nerve plexi of the enteric nervous system and by the extrinsic nerve fibres in the vagus nerve and sympathetic nerves. In general, cholinergic fibres stimulate gastric secretion and motility and adrenergic fibres have the opposite effect, generally inhibiting secretion and motility.

Acetylcholine released from the cholinergic fibres in local nerves stimulates oxyntic (parietal) cells to release acid, or G cells to secrete gastrin. Some fibres in the vagus nerve also contain gastrin releasing peptide (GRP). GRP released from the nerves in the stomach stimulates gastrin release from the G cells. This interaction of the neural and gastrin mechanisms facilitates a rapid response to food ingestion.

Inhibitory control of acid secretion
Gastric acid secretion is blocked if the contents of the stomach become too acidic (pH 3.0 or lower). Inhibition is indirect and is exerted via inhibition of gastrin release. This negative feedback mechanism prevents the gastric and duodenal contents becoming too acidic. If the acidity of the stomach drops below pH 2.0 it is virtually impossible to stimulate gastrin release by any means. Numerous peptides inhibit acid secretion; Figure 4.2 gives a summary of gastrointestinal peptides that inhibit acid production in the stomach.

Other inhibitory factors
The hormone secretin also profoundly inhibits gastrin release and gastric acid secretion. It is released from the duodenum in response to presence of chyme in the first part of the small intestine. The most potent stimulus for secretin release is acid in the duodenum. Secretin inhibits the secretion of gastrin from G cells and the secretion of acid from the oxyntic (parietal) cells. Other peptides that inhibit gastric acid secretion are gastric inhibitory peptide (GIP), released in response to fatty foodstuffs in the duodenum, and vasoactive intestinal peptide (VIP).

Control of pepsinogen secretion
Pepsin is a co-factor in the acid-induced ulceration of the stomach and the duodenum. Its precursor, pepsinogen, is released from the chief cells in response to acetylcholine, as well as by a number of gastrointestinal hormones. Acetylcholine acts upon muscarinic receptors on the chief cell membrane where

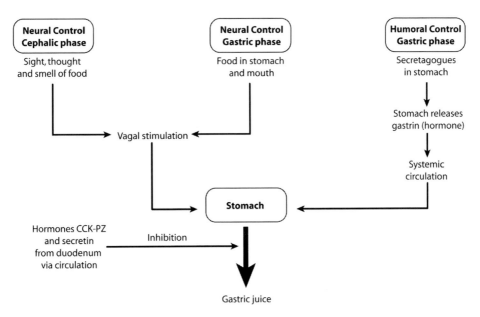

Figure 4.2 Summary of gastrointestinal peptides. Reproduced with permission from Hinchliff *et al.* (1996).

H$^+$ ions stimulate the release of pepsinogen. Gastrin stimulates pepsinogen directly via receptors; however, the most potent effect of gastrin upon pepsinogen secretion is its indirect action via acid secretion.

PATHOPHYSIOLOGY OF THE STOMACH

Pathophysiological conditions that are seen in the stomach include gastritis, gastric and duodenal ulceration and tumours of the stomach.

Gastritis

Gastritis means inflammation of the gastric mucosa. It is caused by irritants, such as gastric acid, bile reflux, medications or toxins. Gastritis is often associated with an impairment of natural protective mechanisms. It can be classified according to its inflammatory pattern as acute (erosive, haemorrhagic gastritis) or chronic (non-erosive gastritis).

Acute gastritis

This may involve the gastric body and antrum of the stomach and is often erosive and haemorrhagic. The response of the gastric mucosa to trauma is similar to that in other tissues with the release of an array of physiologically active substances. Erythema and oedema are predominant features.

Causes of acute gastritis

Acute gastritis often produces no symptoms but may cause dyspepsia, anorexia, nausea or vomiting, haematemesis or melaena. Many cases resolve quickly and do not merit investigation; in others endoscopy and biopsy may be necessary to exclude peptic ulcer, cancer or bleeding. Treatment should be directed to the underlying cause. Acute gastritis almost always responds to conservative therapy with oral antacids.

Chronic gastritis

Chronic gastritis is common in adults and may be associated with a number of conditions including gastric ulcers and *Helicobacter pylori* (HP). It usually involves the gastric body and antrum of the stomach. Most patients are asymptomatic and do not require any treatment. At present there is no indication for widespread use of HP eradication therapy in patients with chronic gastritis but without evidence of peptic ulcer disease.

Chronic gastritis can be classified as:

- Type A (autoimmune)
- Type B (bacterial infection)
- Type C (reflux gastritis)

Type A: autoimmune chronic gastritis (ACG)

ACG involves the body of the stomach but does not affect the antral region and results from autoimmune activity against parietal cells. The histological features are diffuse chronic inflammation, atrophy and loss of fundi glands, intestinal metaplasia and sometimes hyperplasia of enterochromaffin-like (ECL) cells. In some patients the degree of gastric atrophy is severe and loss of intrinsic factor secretion leads to pernicious anaemia. The gastritis itself is usually asymptomatic but some patients have evidence of other organ-specific autoimmunity, particularly thyroid disease. There is a fourfold increase in the risk of gastric cancer development.

Type B: bacterial infection

HP infection is present in about 90% of Type B gastritis cases. It provokes an acute inflammatory response. Type B gastritis can affect the entire stomach.

Type C: reflux gastritis

Reflux gastritis is caused by the regurgitation of duodenal contents into the stomach through the pylorus. It may be present with dyspepsia and bilious vomiting.

Peptic ulcer disease

Duodenal ulcer and gastric ulcer are often grouped together as peptic ulcers. The term 'peptic ulcer' refers to an ulcer in the lower oesophagus, stomach or duodenum. Ulcers in the stomach or duodenum may be acute or chronic; both penetrate the muscularis mucosae but the acute ulcer shows no evidence of fibrosis. Erosions do not penetrate the muscularis mucosae.

When the normal balance is upset between the factors which promote mucosal injury (gastric acid, pepsin, bile acids and ingested substances) and those that protect the mucosa (intact epithelium, mucus lining, bicarbonate secretion), peptic ulceration can occur. The development of ulceration may be mechanical, chemical, infectious or ischaemic in nature. It is thought that in some patients decreased pyloric sphincter pressure may permit the reflux of duodenal material into the stomach; the presence of such material disrupts the gastric mucosal barrier, exposing it to acid. Subsequent histamine release leads to oedema and mucosal erosion.

Clinical features of peptic ulcers

The most common clinical presentation is recurrent abdominal pain, which is localised to the epigastric region, is related to the intake of food and has an episodic pattern.

Pain is referred to the epigastrium and is often so sharply localised that the patient can indicate its site with two or three fingers (the 'pointing sign'). Pain occurs intermittently during the day, often when the stomach is empty, such that the patient identifies it as 'hunger pain' and achieves relief by eating. Night pain is common in duodenal ulceration and can disrupt sleep.

In general, ulcer pain is relieved by food, milk or antacids and by belching and vomiting. Relief by vomiting is more typical of gastric ulcer than of duodenal ulcer; some patients learn to induce vomiting to gain pain relief. Pain is episodic and may last for several weeks at a time. Between episodes the patient feels perfectly well. Other symptoms, especially during episodes of pain, include waterbrash, heartburn, loss of appetite and vomiting. Occasionally the only symptoms are anorexia and nausea, or a sense of undue repletion after meals. In some patients the ulcer is completely 'silent', presenting for the first time with anaemia from chronic undetected blood loss, as an abrupt haematemesis or as acute perforation; in other patients there is recurrent acute bleeding without ulcer pain between the attacks.

Although the prevalence of peptic ulcer is decreasing in many Western communities, it still affects approximately 10% of all adults at some time in their lives. The male to female ratio for duodenal ulcer varies from 5:1 to 2:1, whilst that for a gastric ulcer is 2:1 or less.

Typical risk factors for gastric ulcer disease include the following:

- *Helicobacter pylori* (HP) infection
- chronic usage of non-steroidal anti-inflammatory drugs (NSAIDs)
- familial history of gastric ulceration
- cigarette smoking
- stress and personality type

Helicobacter pylori

In recent years evidence has accumulated that infection of the gastric mucosa by the bacterium *H. pylori* is a causative factor in the development of ulcer disease. These spiral Gram-negative bacteria are found in the stomach of over 80% of patients with gastric or duodenal ulcers. Up to 90% of the population are infected with *H. pylori* by adult life in the Western world. The vast majority of individuals with a presence of the HP bacteria are usually healthy and asymptomatic and only a minority develop clinical disease (www.helico.com accessed 8 May 2004).

Pathophysiolgy of HP infection

The HP bacterium has many flagella attached to one end, making it highly mobile. It has adapted to the acidic nature of the stomach by burrowing beneath the mucosa of the stomach. Here the surface pH is close to neutral and any acidity is buffered by the organism's production of the enzyme urease. Urease produces ammonia from urea and raises the pH around the bacterium. Although it is non-invasive, the bacterium stimulates chronic gastritis by provoking a local inflammatory response in the underlying epithelium due to release of a range of cytotoxins. Once infection in the antrum is established, there is depletion of antral somatostatin and stimulation of gastrin release from G-cells. The subsequent increased flow of blood to the region (hypergastrinaemia) stimulates acid production by the parietal cells, leading to duodenal mucosal damage. Consequences of *H. pylori* infection include gastritis and gastric and duodenal ulcers.

Diagnosis of HP infection

Multiple methods are available for the detection of HP infection. Non-invasive methods include serology for antibody or antigen detection. Invasive procedures include biopsy during endoscopy for histology or rapid urease testing. These procedures are further examined in Chapter 10. For the latest information on HP consult the Heliobacter Foundation (www.helico.com accessed 8 May 2004).

Non-steroidal anti-inflammatory drugs (NSAIDs)

NSAIDs, such as indomethacin and ibuprofen, are effective anti-inflammatory agents which damage the gastric mucosal barrier and are important causal factors in gastric ulcers (Misiewicz and Punder 2000). These drugs also reduce the integrity of the duodenal mucosa but are probably responsible for only a small proportion of duodenal ulcers. They greatly increase the risk of bleeding or perforation from pre-existing gastric and duodenal ulcers.

Risk factors for NSAID-induced ulcers have been identified and should be considered when reviewing a patient's medication, although the availibility of over-the-counter NSAID preparations should be recognised. Risk factors for NSAID-induced ulcers include:

- age > 60 years
- past history of peptic ulcer
- past history of adverse event with NSAIDs
- concurrent use of corticosteroids
- high-dose or multiple NSAIDs

Management of NSAID ulcers
If possible the offending NSAID drug should be discontinued. If an NSAID must be used then one with a lower risk of complications, e.g. ibuprofen, should be used at the lowest effective dose. Co-prescription of a proton pump inhibitor will heal most, but not all, ulcers.

Heredity

Patients with peptic ulcer often have a family history of ulcers, particularly in the case of duodenal ulcers in individuals under the age of 20. Links with blood group O and non-secretor status have been observed but the pathogenic significance of these findings is uncertain.

Smoking

Smoking gives an increased risk of gastric ulcer and, to a lesser extent, duodenal ulcer. Once the ulcer has formed it is more likely to cause complications and less likely to heal on standard treatment regimens if smoking continues. Individuals with gastric ulceration should be encouraged to cease smoking.

Acid-pepsin versus mucosal resistance

An ulcer forms when there is an imbalance between aggressive factors, i.e. from the digestive power of gastric acid and pepsin, and defensive factors, i.e. the ability of the gastric and duodenal mucosa to resist this digestive power. This mucosal resistance constitutes the gastric mucosal barrier. Ulcers occur only in the presence of acid and pepsin; they are never found in achlorhydric patients such as those with pernicious anaemia. On the other hand, severe intractable peptic ulceration nearly always occurs in patients with Zollinger-Ellison syndrome, which is characterised by very high acid secretion.

Investigation of peptic ulcer

Diagnosis can be made by double-contrast barium meal examination or by endoscopic investigation. Endoscopy is the preferred investigation because it is more accurate and has the enormous advantage that suspicious lesions and HP status can be concurrently evaluated by biopsy. For those with a duodenal ulcer seen at barium meal, urea breath testing will accurately define the HP status. In gastric ulcer disease endoscopy must be repeated after suitable treatment to confirm that the ulcer has healed.

Management of peptic ulcer disease

HP eradication is the cornerstone of modern therapy for peptic ulcers, as this will successfully prevent relapse and eliminate the need for long-term therapy in the majority of patients. All patients with proven acute or chronic duodenal ulcer disease, and those with gastric ulcers who are HP-positive, should be offered eradication therapy as first-line treatment. Treatment is based upon a proton pump inhibitor taken simultaneously with two antibiotics for a period of seven days. Compliance, side-effects and metronidazole resistance influence the success of therapy.

Nurses involved in the care of patients with peptic ulcer disease may include behavioural modification techniques by incorporating the following recommendations:

- Cease smoking.
- NSAIDs should be avoided.
- Alcohol should be taken in moderation.
- No specific dietary advice is required.

At present, the most frequently used medical treatment for the suppression of gastric acid secretion in peptic ulcer disease is the administration of proton pump inhibitors. These inhibitors are effective in decreasing gastric acid by inhibiting the enzyme responsible for the final step of acid secretion, hydrogen-potassium adenosinetriphosphatase (ATPase) in the parietal cell membrane. After a few days of treatment, virtual achlorhydria is achieved and rapid healing of both gastric and duodenal ulcers follows. Omeprazole and lansoprazole are important components of HP eradication regimens. Proton pump inhibitors are also much more effective than H2 antagonists for the healing and maintenance of reflux oesophagitis.

Other drugs available for the short-term management of peptic ulcer symptoms and other dyspeptic disorders include antacids and histamine H_2 receptor antagonists. These can be purchased without prescription in the UK.

Antacids act to neutralise gastric acid and strengthen the gastric mucosal barrier. They are widely available for self-medication and are used for relief of minor dyspeptic symptoms. Calcium compounds cause constipation, while magnesium-containing agents cause diarrhoea.

Reduction of acid secretion in peptic ulcer disease can be effected by antagonising the action of histamine. Using histamine H_2 receptor antagonists, symptoms remit promptly, usually within days of starting treatment, and 80% of duodenal ulcers will heal after four weeks. These drugs do not inhibit acid secretion to the same degree as the proton pump inhibitors but are useful for the short-term management of reflux oesophagitis.

The effectiveness of diet manipulation in ulcer healing is unknown. Foods known to increase acid secretion include milk, alcohol and coffee.

Surgical management of peptic ulcer disease
Surgery was once the definitive treatment for peptic ulcer disease. However, the development of effective acid-suppressing drugs has made elective surgery for peptic ulcer disease a rare event. Emergency gastric surgery is indicated for patients who do not adhere to medical therapy, and for peptic ulcers which are refractive to medical therapy, or in extreme circumstances of uncontrolled haemorrhage from a gastric ulcer. Three surgical procedures are indicated for the treatment of peptic ulcer disease: partial gastrectomy with gastroduodenostomy, partial gastrectomy with gastrojejunostomy, and highly selective vagotomy.

Complications of peptic ulcer disease

The main complications of peptic ulcer disease are perforation, gastric outlet obstruction and bleeding.

Perforation
When perforation occurs, the contents of the stomach escape into the peritoneal cavity, leading to peritonitis. Perforation occurs more commonly in duodenal than in gastric ulcers, and usually in ulcers on the anterior wall.

Although perforation may be the first sign of an ulcer, there is commonly a history of recurrent epigastric pain. The most striking symptom is sudden, severe pain; its distribution follows the spread of the gastric contents over the peritoneum. Pain initially develops in the upper abdomen and rapidly becomes degeneralised; shoulder tip pain is due to irritation of the diaphragm. The pain is accompanied by shallow respiration due to limitation of diaphragmatic movements, and by shock. The abdomen is held immobile and there is generalised 'board-like' rigidity. Vomiting is common. After some hours symptoms improve, although abdominal rigidity remains. Later the patient's condition deteriorates as general peritonitis develops.

After initial resuscitation the acute perforation is usually treated surgically, either by simple closure or by closure combined with vagotomy and drainage. Patients who are found to be HP-positive should undergo eradication therapy. Perforation is more common in men and the outlook is worst for older patients with large perforations (Misiewicz and Punder 2000).

Gastric outlet obstruction
Another complication of peptic ulcer disease is gastric outlet obstruction. Obstruction of the pyloric sphincter at the outlet of the stomach blocks the flow of gastric contents into the duodenum. Nausea, vomiting, gastric pain and abdominal distension are the cardinal features of such obstruction. The gastric pain is aggravated by eating and many patients with gastric outlet

obstruction may become anorexic. Loss of gastric contents leads to dehydration with low serum sodium, chloride and potassium, and raised bicarbonate and urea concentrations. Nasogastric aspiration of food residue or at least 200 ml of fluid from the stomach after an overnight fast suggests the diagnosis.

Endoscopy should be performed after the stomach has been emptied by a wide-bore nasogastric tube in order to confirm or refute organic obstruction. Barium studies are rarely advisable because they cannot usually distinguish between peptic ulcer or cancer. Moreover, barium remains in the stomach and is difficult to remove.

Treatment begins with restoration of fluid and electrolyte balance, correction of nutritional deficiences and decompression of the stomach. Nasogastric suction and intravenous correction of dehydration and metabolic acidosis are undertaken. In some patients ulcer healing with proton pump inhibitors relieves pyloric oedema and surgery is not required. In other patients vagotomy and gastroenterostomy are necessary, although they are best carried out after seven days of gastric aspiration, which enables the stomach to return to normal size.

Gastrointestinal bleeding
Peptic ulceration is the leading cause of upper gastrointestinal bleeding, accounting for half of all cases. The specific nursing management of patients with an upper gastrointestinal bleed is addressed in Chapter 11.

Stress ulcers

Stress ulcers are gastric mucosal stress erosions that are associated with a serious illness. They appear to be associated with the following situations:

- severe trauma
- extreme burns
- intracranial trauma (Cushing's ulcer)
- gastric erosive drugs

The only symptom of a stress ulcer is an upper gastrointestinal bleed. Treatment in stress ulcers is focused upon control of the bleeding, correcting the shock and treating the underlying disorder.

Zollinger-Ellison syndrome

In this rare disorder a gastrin secreting neuroendocrine tumour of the pancreas ('gastrinoma') is present with recurrent duodenal ulceration and diarrhoea. It accounts for only about 0.1% of all cases of duodenal ulceration (Misiewicz and Punder 2000). The syndrome occurs in either sex at any age, although it is most common between 30 and 50 years. Patients with Zollinger-Ellison syndrome present with pain as the predominant symptom from peptic ulcer disease; they also have diarrhoea and steatorrhoea.

Peptic ulcers are often multiple and severe and there is a poor response to standard ulcer medical therapy. The history is usually short; bleeding and perforations are common.

Pathophysiology of Zollinger-Ellison syndrome
Tumours mostly occur in the pancreatic head or tail (Misiewicz and Punder 2000). The gastrinoma secretes large amounts of gastrin, which stimulates the parietal cells of the stomach to secrete acid to their maximal capacity and increases the parietal cell mass three to sixfold. The acid output may be so great that it reaches the upper small intestine, reducing the luminal pH to 2 or less. Pancreatic lipase is inactivated and bile acids are precipitated.

An increased serum gastrin is the most specific and reliable test for Zollinger-Ellinson syndrome. Gastrin levels are grossly elevated (ten to one thousand-fold). Tumour localisation is often attempted using a CT scan.

Management of Zollinger-Ellison syndrome
Approximately 30% of small and single tumours can be localised and resected but many tumours are multifocal. Some patients present with metastatic disease and surgery is inappropriate. Advances in medical treatment have made total gastrectomy unnecessary, and in the majority of patients continuous therapy with proton pump inhibitors heals ulcers and alleviates diarrhoea. Larger doses (60–80 mg daily) than those used to treat duodenal ulcer are required.

Functional disorders of the stomach

Non-ulcer dyspepsia (functional dyspepsia)

Symptoms that mimic an ulcer in patients who have no objective evidence of an ulcer are termed non-ulcer dyspepsia. Dyspepsia is a rather vague term that relates to symptoms of epigastric discomfort, burning or pain, nausea, bloating and belching. The condition of non-ulcer dyspepsia probably covers a spectrum of mucosal, motility and psychiatric disorders. The symptoms caused by motor dysfunction are analogous to the motility disturbances that occur in irritable bowel syndrome; indeed, these disorders commonly occur together.

Clinical features of non-ulcer dyspepsia
In general, patients are usually young (< 40 years) and women are affected more than men. Abdominal pain is associated with a variable combination of other 'dyspeptic' symptoms, the commonest being nausea and bloating after meals. Morning symptoms are characteristic and pain or nausea may occur on waking. Direct enquiry may elicit symptoms suggestive of colonic dysmotility, such as pellet-like stools or a sense of incomplete rectal evacuation on defaecation. Peptic ulcer disease must be considered, whilst in older subjects intra-abdominal malignancy is a prime concern.

Symptoms may appear disproportionate to clinical well-being and there is no weight loss. Patients often appear anxious and distraught and it is sometimes possible to detect psychological symptoms. A drug history should be taken and the possibility of psychological morbidity should be considered in nursing assessment. In many cases a simple history will often suggest the diagnosis but in older subjects an endoscopy is necessary to exclude mucosal disease.

Management of non-ulcer dyspepsia

Explanation and reassurance are essential for patients with non-ulcer dyspepsia. Possible psychological factors should be explored and the concept of psychological influences on gut function should be explained. Lifestyle advice may be necessary; cigarette smoking and alcohol abuse should be discouraged and sensible dietary advice provided.

Drug treatment should only be used when symptoms are intolerable. Antacids are sometimes helpful. Prokinetic drugs, such as metoclopramide or cisapride, may be given before meals if nausea, vomiting or bloating are prominent. H_2-receptor antagonist drugs may be tried if night pain or heartburn are troublesome. Symptoms which can be associated with an identifiable cause of stress may resolve with appropriate nursing support or counselling. Some patients have major chronic psychological disorders resulting in persistent or recurrent symptoms and may require formal psychotherapy.

Evidence-based guidelines for the management of non-ulcer dyspepsia have been written by Vakil (2001).

Vomiting

Vomiting is part of the protective role of the stomach as it protects the body from the ingestion of toxic substances. This role augments the other main protective mechanisms of the stomach, acid and pepsin secretion and mucin secretion, which protect the columnar epithelium.

Vomiting or emesis is the forceful ejection of gastric contents and sometimes duodenal contents, through the mouth. It is a reflex which is usually preceded by a feeling of nausea. Vomiting is usually accompanied by salivation, sweating, pallor, a fall in blood pressure, increased heart rate and irregular breathing. The vomiting reflex is controlled by the vomiting centre in the medulla oblongata and the reflex involves stimulation of the respiratory and abdominal skeletal muscles as well as the smooth muscle of the gastrointestinal tract.

Psychogenic vomiting may occur in anxiety neurosis. It starts usually on wakening, or immediately after breakfast; only rarely does it occur later in the day. The disorder is probably a reaction to facing up to the worries of everyday life, for example in the young it can be due to school phobia. There may be retching alone or the vomiting of gastric secretions or food. Although psychogenic vomiting may occur regularly over long periods, there is little or no weight loss.

In all patients it is essential to address any underlying psychological circumstances. Tranquilisers and anti-emetic drugs have only a secondary place in the management of a patient with vomiting.

Tumours of the stomach

Gastric carcinoma

Gastric cancer is exceptional, in that its incidence has been declining for the past 20 years whilst other gastrointestinal tumours have increased in frequency. Despite this, it remains a common cause of death in the Western world and is extremely common in China, Japan and parts of South America. Variations in populations are believed to be due to local environmental, mainly dietary, factors. Gastric cancer is more common in men and the incidence rises sharply after 50 years of age. Ninety-seven per cent of gastric cancers are adenocarcinomas; the remaining 3% are lymphomas, carcinoid tumours or sarcomas (Clark *et al.* 2000).

Helicobacter pylori, which is known to predispose to peptic ulcer disease, has also been linked to gastric carcinoma. HP infection may be responsible for 60–70% of cases and acquisition of infection at an early age may be important. Although the majority of HP-infected individuals have normal or increased acid secretion, a few become hypo- or achlorhydric and these people are thought to be at greatest risk (www.helico.com accessed 8 May 2004).

Recognised dietary factors associated with gastric carcinoma include foods that are rich in salted, smoked or pickled foods (such as vegetables, fish and meat) and the consumption of nitrites and nitrates are also associated with cancer risk. Carcinogenic N-nitroso-compounds are formed from nitrates by the action of nitrite-reducing bacteria which colonise the achlorhydric stomach. A diet which is lacking in fresh fruit and vegetables as well as vitamins A and C may also be a contributing factor. Other recognised risk factors include smoking and heavy alcohol intake.

The clinical signs and symptoms of gastric cancer include epigastric discomfort, vomiting and presence of faecal occult blood. Depending on the location of the lesion, patients can present with a variety of symptoms including:

- unexplained weight loss
- early satiety or anorexia
- anaemia
- abdominal mass
- gastric outlet obstruction
- vomiting and nausea
- ascites
- enlarged lymph nodes

Examination may reveal no abnormalities, but signs of weight loss, anaemia or a palpable epigastric mass are not infrequent. Jaundice or ascites may signify metastatic spread. Occasionally tumour spread occurs to the supraclavicular lymph nodes, umbilicus or ovaries. Metastases occur most commonly in the liver, lungs, peritoneum, bone and marrow.

Most adenocarcinomas arise from mucus-secreting cells in the base of the gastric crypts. Most develop on a background of chronic atrophic gastritis with intestinal metaplasia and dysplasia.

Approximately half of all gastric cancers occur in the antral region of the stomach and 20–30% are situated in the gastric body, often on the greater curve (Clark *et al.* 2000). About 20% occur in the cardia and this type of tumour is becoming more common.

Early gastric cancer is defined as cancer confined to the mucosa or submucosa, regardless of lymph node involvement. It is often recognised in Japan, where widespread use of endoscopic screening is practised. Most patients in the Western world present with advanced gastric cancer.

Diagnosis and staging of gastric cancer
Gastric cancer may be diagnosed by upper gastrointestinal endoscopy, CT (computerised tomography) scan, plain stomach or chest X-ray films and double-contrast upper gastrointestinal series. Upper gastrointestinal endoscopy is the investigation of choice and should be performed promptly in any patient with 'alarm symptoms' such as unexplained weight loss, rectal bleeding and a family history of gastric carcinoma. Once the diagnosis is made, further imaging is necessary for accurate staging and assessment of the tumour for resectability. Endoscopic ultrasound will demonstrate whether the lesion has penetrated the submucosa or not and will also allow for visualisation of infiltrated lymph nodes. CT scans may not demonstrate small involved lymph nodes, but will show evidence of intra-abdominal spread or liver metastases. Even with these techniques, laparoscopy may be required to determine whether the tumour is resectable.

Treatment of gastric cancer
Surgery is the treatment of choice for curable lesions. Unfortunately many gastric cancers present at an advanced stage; patients may have an enlarged liver and associated jaundice – due to blood-borne metastases. Treatment for advanced cancer is largely palliative. It involves surgical resection of the tumour to relieve obstruction or dysphagia, or to control chronic bleeding. Following surgery, combination chemotherapy may be used alone or in conjunction with localised radiotherapy. Complications of gastric cancer, such as perforation and obstruction, should be managed as and when they occur.

Carcinomas at the cardia of the stomach may require endoscopic dilation, laser therapy or insertion of expandable metallic stents to allow adequate swallowing.

There are many nursing responsibilities in the care of the patient with a terminal illness including: meeting the emotional needs of the individual, providing adequate nutrition, and management of the patient's pain.

Resection offers the only hope of cure and this can be achieved in 80–90% of patients with early gastric cancer. For the majority of patients who present with locally advanced disease, tumours of the distal stomach require partial gastrectomy, while cancers of the proximal body or cardia may require oesophagogastrectomy. Extensive lymph node resection may also increase survival rates but carries greater morbidity. Even for those who cannot be cured, palliative resection may be safely performed in patients with low morbidity and may be necessary if features such as gastric outlet obstruction are present.

Prognosis
Apart from patients with early gastric cancer the prognosis remains very poor, with less than 10% surviving five years (Clark *et al.* 2000). Even after an apparently curative resection, five-year survival is only around 20%. Thus the best hope for improved survival lies in greater detection of tumours at an earlier stage. The low incidence of gastric carcinoma in many Western countries makes widespread endoscopic screening impractical, but urgent referral and investigation of patients with new-onset dyspepsia over the age of 45, or those with 'alarm' symptoms, is essential.

Evidence-based guidelines for the management of gastric cancer have been published by Allum *et al.* (2002).

Gastric polyps

Gastric polyps are defined as any restricted, discrete stomach tumour and they are relatively uncommon. They develop most often after the age of 55. Gastric polyps are more common in patients with achlorhydria, atrophic gastric, pernicious anaemia or gastric cancer, or patients who have undergone gastric resection. Unless a polyp bleeds it does not usually cause symptoms. Gastric polyps are usually detected on endoscopy and are treated by endoscopic polypectomy.

Conclusion

The stomach plays a crucial role in digestion by breaking down food into particles which are sufficiently small to continue the journey through the remainder of the digestive tract. This mechanical breakdown also increases the surface area of the food available for chemical breakdown, which is initiated in the stomach by the release of the enzyme pepsin. The stomach also acts as an effective 'acid bath' achieving very high acidity and thereby killing most pathogens which may be ingested. However, the digestive functions of the stomach, which mainly rely on the high acidity in the stomach, can also lead to problems when things go wrong. The stomach has an effective defence against the high acidity of its contents, which would corrode other tissues of the body, in the shape of the copious mucus, which is also secreted by the stomach. When this mucus becomes disrupted or deficient, the stomach wall itself is left vulnerable to corrosion by its acidic contents. The acid contents of the stomach can, as we have seen, cause problems in the oesophagus, which leads to the stomach, and also in the duodenum, which receives the contents of the stomach as they enter the small intestine. The control of digestion in the stomach is initiated by the presence or even the thought of food; the stomach partly controls digestion itself and the presence of food in the intestine also exerts control.

The disorders of the stomach are all in some way related to the acidity of the stomach contents. These disorders range from the discomfort of gastritis through the pain and potential threat to life of ulcerative conditions. Cancer of the stomach may share some of the aetiology of the ulcerative conditions in that the *Helicobacter pylori* bacterium is associated with it.

In common with the disorders of the oesophagus, disorders of the stomach often require endoscopic examination, among other procedures. The performance of these procedures and the outcome for the patients are often distressing and nurses have a major role to play in explaining to the patient what is going to happen and accompanying them during any investigations. The options for disorders of the stomach – depending upon the diagnosis – range from drug therapy to major surgery, therefore the patient with a disorder of the stomach will require considerable support from nursing staff, including information to reinforce the medical diagnosis and, where appropriate, advice about lifestyle change. In the case of advanced stomach cancer a realistic assessment of the outcome of surgery will need to be reinforced, with attention paid to the significant others of the patient.

BACKGROUND READING

Additional reading to support the material in this chapter can be found in the relevant sections of the following texts:

Alexander, M., Fawcett, J.N. and Runciman, P. (2000) *Nursing Practice: Hospital and Home – the Adult.* Churchill Livingstone, Edinburgh (Chapter 4).

Brooker, C. and Nicol, M. (2003) *Nursing Adults: the Practice of Caring.* Mosby, London (Chapter 22).

Clancy, J. and McVicar, A.J. (2002) *Physiology and Anatomy: a Homeostatic Approach*, 2nd edition. Arnold, London (Chapter 10).

Clancy, J., McVicar, A.J. and Baird, N. (2002) *Perioperative Practice: Fundamentals of Homeostasis.* Routledge, London (Chapter 2).

Haslett, C., Chilvers, E.R., Boon, N.A. and Colledge, N.R. (2002) *Davidson's Principles and Practice of Medicine*, 19th edition. Churchill Livingstone, Edinburgh (Chapter 17).

Hinchliff, S., Montague, S. and Watson, R. (1996) *Physiology for Nursing Practice*, 2nd edition. Baillière Tindall, London (Chapter 5.1).

Kindlen, S. (2003) *Physiology for Health Care and Nursing.* Churchill Livingstone, Edinburgh (Chapter 20).

Kumar, P. and Clark, M. (2002) *Clinical Medicine*, 4th edition. Saunders, Edinburgh (Chapter 6).

McKenry, L.M. and Salerno, E. (1998) *Pharmacology for Nursing*, 20th edition. Mosby, St Louis (Unit 11).
Watson, R. (2000) *Anatomy and Physiology for Nurses*, 11th edition. Baillière Tindall, London (Chapter 20).

EVIDENCE-BASED GUIDELINES

Allum, W.H., Griffin, S.M., Watson, A. and Colin-Jones, D. (2002) Guidelines for the management of oesophageal and gastric cancer. *Gut*, **50**, Suppl V, v1–v23 (http://www.bsg.org.uk/pdf_word_docs/ogcancer.pdf accessed 8 May 2004).
Vakil, N. (2001) Dyspepsia, non-ulcer dyspepsia and *Helicobacter pylori*. *Reviews in Gastroenterological Disorders*, **1**, 139–146 (http://www.medreviews.com/pdfs/articles/RIGD_13_139.pdf accessed 8 May 2004).

REFERENCES

Clark, M.L., Talbot, I.C., Thomas, H.J.W. and Williams, C.B. (2000) Tumours of the gastrointestinal tract. In: *Concise Oxford Textbook of Medicine* (Leadingham, J.G.G. and Worrell, D.A., eds), pp. 577–84. Oxford University Press, Oxford.
Misiewicz, J.J. and Punder, R.E. (2000) Peptic ulceration. In: *Concise Oxford Textbook of Medicine* (Leadingham, J.G.G. and Worrell, D.A., eds), pp. 530–37. Oxford University Press, Oxford.

Chapter 5
The Small Intestine

Chapter objectives

After reading this chapter you should be able to:

- Describe the anatomy and physiology of the small intestine.
- Understand the physiology of intestinal absorption, secretion and motility.
- Identify the major disorders of the small intestine.
- Relate the pathophysiology, diagnosis and treatment of disorders of the small intestine to nursing care.

ANATOMY AND PHYSIOLOGY

The small intestine is a convoluted tube, with two concentric layers of smooth muscle, that extends from the pyloric sphincter to its junction with the large intestine at the ileo-caecal valve. It is approximately 6 m long with a 3.5 cm diameter and lies in the central and lower part of the abdominal cavity. The small intestines consist of three sections:

- duodenum
- jejunum
- ileum

The first 30 cm of the small intestine is the C-shaped muscular duodenum, which begins at the pyloric sphincter in the stomach. The common bile duct empties into the duodenum at the ampulla of vater.

After the duodenum, the proximal two-fifths of the small bowel (2.5 m) is known as the jejunum. The distal three-fifths of the small intestine, known as the ileum (3.5 m), extends from the jejunum to the ileo-caecal valve. This important physiological valve controls the flow of chyme into the large intestine and prevents backflow or reflux into the small intestine. No anatomical feature separates the jejunum from the ileum and their structure is consistent with that of the duodenum.

The surface of the duodenum is folded. These folds are known as plicae circulares (circular folds). However, there is a gradual decease in the diameter, thickness of the wall and number of folds, with distance from the duodenum. The folds are virtually absent in the terminal portion of the ileum. The mucosa of the small intestine is covered with tiny projections, known as villi. These villi become less numerous, smaller and more finger-like with distance from the duodenum. Numerous lymphatic nodes, called Peyer's patches, are present in the mucosa and submucosa in the ileum. These are circular, aggregated lymph nodes that participate in the body's immune response and synthesise antibodies.

The terminal junction of the ileum joins the large intestine at the ileo-caecal valve. It is approximately 4 cm long in an adult and consists of a ring of thickened smooth muscle. Relaxation and contraction of this sphincter controls the rate of entry of chyme into the colon. The ileo-caecal valve may also have an important role in preventing the movement of bacteria from the large bowel into the ileum. This sphincter is normally closed, but when peristalsis takes place in the terminal ileum, distension of the region causes a reflex relaxation of the sphincter muscle. This allows a small amount of chyme to enter the large intestine. The rate of entry into the colon is appropriately slow to allow salt and water absorption from the chyme before the next portion of chyme enters.

The wall of the small intestine is composed of the following layers:

- Serosa: an outer layer composed of peritoneum and connective tissue.
- Muscularis: containing outer longitudinal and inner circular layers of muscle, separated by the myenteric plexus nerve network.
- Submucosa: connective tissue, which contains blood vessels, lymphatic tissue and a submucosal nerve plexus.
- Mucosa: inner mucosa layer.

The surface of the small intestine forms a series of circular folds which increase the surface area available for absorption of nutrients. The surface has a velvety appearance owing to the presence of fine hair-like projections called villi, each containing a lymph vessel (lacteal) and blood vessels. Each villus is lined with simple columnar epithelial cells. Below the epithelium the lamina propria separates the mucosa from the submucosa. A brush border consisting of multiple microvilli covers the surface of each columnar cell. The mucosa is supplied with simple, tubular-type glands which secrete intestinal juice.

The villus is regarded as a unit of absorption. Its length can vary between 0.5 and 1 mm, depending on the location in the small intestine. The structure of the villus is shown in Figure 5.1. Each villus contains a blood capillary network and a blind-ended lacteal, which is a lymph vessel. The villus is covered by simple columnar epithelium. Most of these cells have numerous cytoplasmic extensions at the luminal surface, known as microvilli. The microvillus surface

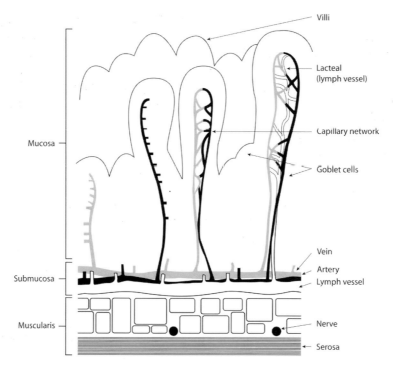

Figure 5.1 Structure of the villus. Reproduced with permission from Hinchliff *et al.*
(1996).

of the small intestine is known as the brush border. The presence of the mucosal
folds, the villi and the microvilli increases the surface area and therefore the
absorptive capacity of the small bowel by approximately five hundredfold.

The mucosa of the small intestine is simple columnar epithelium. Four major cell types are present:

- Absorptive cells, which produce digestive enzymes and absorb nutrients
  from digested food.
- Goblet cells, which produce protective mucus that lubricates the surface
  and protects it from mechanical damage.
- Granular cells, which protect the intestinal epithelium from bacteria.
- Endocrine cells, which produce peptide hormones that regulate secretion
  and motility in the gastrointestinal tract, liver and pancreas.

Two types of gland are present in the duodenum. At the base of the villi are
tubular invaginations that reach almost to the muscularis layer; these are known
as the intestinal crypts or crypts of Lieberkuhn. The submucosa of the duodenum contains coiled compound tubular mucous glands, known as the glands
of Brunner, which secrete an alkaline fluid rich in mucus. These are more
numerous in the proximal region of the duodenum.

Blood supply to the small intestine

The duodenum receives arterial blood from the hepatic artery, whereas the rest of the small intestine blood is derived from the superior mesenteric artery. Numerous arterial branches form an extensive network in the submucosal layer, which supplies the wall of the small intestine. Venous blood from the entire small bowel drains through the superior mesenteric vein.

Nerves, hormones and local paracrine factors control the intestinal circulation. Stimulation of sympathetic nerves causes vasoconstriction and reduced blood flow, enabling a redistribution of blood away from the small intestine. In the blood vessels of the villi, this vasoconstriction effect is short-lived owing to the presence of vasodilator metabolites, such as adenosine, which accumulate during the vasoconstrictor response. Blood flow to the small intestine increases by 50–300% during ingestion of food and this is termed functional hyperaemia. Distension of the small intestine walls and substances present in chyme also stimulate blood flow.

Absorption in the small intestine

The primary function of the small intestine is the absorption of nutrients from chyme. It receives up to eight litres of chyme per day and passes only 500–1000 ml to the large intestine. The remaining fluid is absorbed by the columnar cells of the villous epithelium. Most substances are absorbed in the proximal small intestine. The duodenum is the primary site of iron and calcium absorption, and the jejunum is the site where absorption of fats, carbohydrates and proteins takes place. Finally, only a few substances such as vitamin B_{12} and bile salts are actively absorbed in the ileum. There are a number of barriers to transport from the intestinal lumen to the blood: the luminal plasma membrane, the cell's interior, the intercellular space, the basement membrane of the capillary and the cell membranes of the endothelial cell of the capillary or lymphatic vessels.

There are five basic mechanisms for absorption to take place effectively in the small intestine: hydrolysis, non-ionic movement, passive diffusion, facilitated diffusion and active transport.

Absorption of water in the small intestine

Water transport in the gastrointestinal tract is largely a function of the small intestine. It is an example of passive diffusion across the wall of the small intestine. The stomach is almost impermeable to water but the small intestine is highly permeable; therefore the transport of water in the small intestine can occur both from the lumen to the blood, or from the blood to the lumen. Net transport of water is achieved by the osmotic gradient and it will occur in whatever direction the osmotic forces dictate. Water will be secreted into the lumen if the chyme is hypertonic to the plasma, and absorbed into the blood if it is hypotonic. The chyme entering the duodenum from the pylorus of the stomach is normally hypertonic in nature.

Absorption of electrolytes in the small intestine

Sodium is absorbed along the length of the small bowel but mainly in the jejunum via active transport. Magnesium, phosphate and potassium are absorbed throughout the small intestine.

Absorption of most water-soluble vitamins takes place by diffusion. The exception is vitamin B_{12}, which combines with intrinsic factor (produced by the parietal cells in the stomach) for active transport and is mainly absorbed in the terminal ileum.

Carbohydrates are broken down by digestive enzymes in the intestine into simple sugars (glucose, galactose and fructose), which are then absorbed into the bloodstream via the intestinal mucosa, using either active transport or facilitated diffusion. Proteins are hydrolysed by proteolytic digestive enzymes into amino acids, which are absorbed by active transport.

Fats are emulsified and then broken down into glycerol, fatty acids and glycerides, primarily by the enzyme pancreatic lipase.

Control of absorption in the small intestine

Various factors are involved in the control of water and electrolyte absorption by the cells near the tip of the villi. These include endocrine, paracrine and nervous influences. Glucocorticoids stimulate electrolyte and water absorption in both the small and large intestines. Somatostatin stimulates electrolyte and water absorption in the ileum. Absorption can be inhibited by inflammatory mediators such as histamine and prostaglandins, which are released from cells of the gastrointestinal immune system.

Intestinal secretion

In addition to the absorptive functions of the small intestine, the cells of the small intestine secrete digestive juices, mucus and a variety of hormones. This alkaline intestinal juice contains electrolytes, mucus and water and is secreted throughout the length of the small intestine. The small intestine also receives a variety of secretions from the pancreas and the liver.

The microvilli on the brush border contain the peptidases and disaccharides that are required for digestion of proteins and carbohydrates. Brunner's glands, which are located in the proximal duodenum, secrete a clear, alkaline (pH 8.2–9.0), viscous fluid that acts as a protective layer from gastric acid secretions in the duodenal mucosa. Goblet cells located on and between the villi on the mucosal lining secrete a protective mucus.

Between two and three litres of watery fluid are produced by the crypts of Lieberkuhn each day. This fluid contains a carrier substance for the absorption of nutrients when chyme comes in contact with the villi. There are a variety of endocrine cells located in these crypts, which produce a number of peptides and hormones, including cholecystokinin, secretin, gastrin inhibitory peptide, somatastatin, vasoactive intestinal peptide and serotonin.

Control of intestinal secretions

Secretion in the small intestine can be controlled by hormones, paracrine factors and nervous activity. Hormones and paracrine factors such as gastrin, serotonin and prostaglandins stimulate the epithelial cells directly. The cells are innervated by secretomotor neurones, mainly the ganglia in the submucosal plexus, but also via ganglia in the myenteric plexus. The submucosal neurones release acetylcholine, vasoactive inhibitory peptide and serotonin, to stimulate secretion.

Parasympathetic nerves innervate nerves in the enteric nerve plexi. They enhance secretion by releasing acetylcholine onto the neurones in the plexi. Parasympathetic tone contributes to the basal secretion in the small intestine.

Reflexes triggered by distension of the small intestinal lumen, and the presence of various substances (i.e. glucose, bile salts, acid, alcohol) in the intestinal chyme, stimulate secretion.

There are two ways that noradrenalin has an inhibitory effect upon intestinal secretion. First, it acts directly upon the epithelial cells, and second it acts upon the neurones in the submucosal ganglia to inhibit secretory nerves that stimulate the epithelial cells.

Motility in the small intestine

The smooth muscle lining the small intestine performs two functions. First, it is responsible for a thorough mixing of digestive juices arriving from the pancreas and liver via the common bile duct with the chyme received from the stomach. Second, it is responsible for moving the contents, usually slowly but occasionally rapidly, along the 6 m from the stomach to the ileo-caecal valve. This movement enables one meal to make way for the next. It is vitally important that food is retained in each part of the small intestine for sufficient time to allow for mixing, digestion and absorption of food.

Within the small bowel, three types of movement contribute to the mixing of chyme:

- Concentric, segmenting contractions. Segmentation helps to mix the secretions of the small intestine with the chyme particles.
- Peristaltic waves or short, propulsive contractions. These slowly push the chyme in the direction of the ileo-caecal valve. Peristaltic waves are strongest in the proximal portion of the small bowel.

- The continuous shortening and lengthening of the villi constantly stirs the intestinal contents.

As chyme approaches the large bowel, contractions in the ileum increase.

Control of motility in the small intestine

Motility in the small intestine is under physiological control via several factors, including stretch, extrinsic autonomic nerves, intrinsic nerves of the intramural plexi paracrine factors and circulating hormones.

Neural control of motility in the small intestine
Activation of the intrinsic nerves in the intramural plexi can control segmentation and short peristaltic waves by influencing the basal electrical rhythm, in the absence of hormones or extrinsic nerves. Segmentation and peristalsis are increased by activation of parasympathetic nerves, and inhibited by stimulation of sympathetic nerves. Activation of the sympathetic nervous system, in response to stress for example, results in the release of adrenalin into the circulation, which inhibits intestinal motility. Sympathetic activation also results in vasoconstriction of the blood vessels in the small intestine.

There are many other transmitters, in addition to acetylcholine and catecholamines (adrenalin and noradrenalin), which can influence motility in the small bowel. These include peptides, amines and nucleotides. The peptides include vasoactive intestinal peptide and somatostatin.

Hormonal control of motility in the small intestine
Gastrin, which is released into the blood in response to the presence of peptides in the stomach, and secretin and cholecystokinin, released into the blood in response to the presence of fats and acids in intestinal chyme, all increase intestinal motility. Motilin, a peptide released from the walls of the small intestine into the blood when the intestinal chyme becomes alkaline, increases intestinal motility. Another peptide which is released in the presence of chyme in the small intestine is enteroglucagon. It is released in response to particles of glucose and fat in the chyme. This hormone inhibits peristalsis, and its role allows additional time for absorption of glucose and fat before the chyme reaches the ileo-caecal valve.

Reflex control of motility in the small intestine
Activation of pressure receptors by the distension of the intestinal walls is involved in the reflex control of intestinal motility. A bolus of food placed in the small intestine will cause smooth muscle behind it to contract, and in front of it to relax. When food is present in the stomach, motility increases in the ileum and the ileo-caecal sphincter relaxes. This is known as the gastro-ileal reflex. This reflex appears to be mainly under the control of external nerves

to the mucosa of the intestine; however, gastrin released into the blood in response to chyme in the stomach may augment this reflex.

PATHOPHYSIOLOGY OF THE SMALL BOWEL

The presence of pathological conditions in the small intestine can affect absorption of nutrients of the affected region. It is therefore important to consider the location of the disease to understand fully the impact it can have upon nutrient absorption. Duodenal disease may result in deficiencies of calcium and iron, whereas a diseased jejunum can reduce absorption of fats, carbohydrates and proteins. Vitamin B_{12} deficiency and bile acid malabsorption can result in ileal disease.

Important pathological conditions of the small intestine that will be considered in this section include duodenal ulcer disease, bacterial and viral infections, Crohn's disease, vitamin B_{12} deficiency, small bowel carcinomas and malabsorptive conditions, including coeliac disease.

Duodenal ulcers

Peptic ulcers can develop in the oesophagus, stomach or duodenum. Around 80% of all peptic ulcers are duodenal ulcers (Misiewicz and Punder 2000). Duodenal ulcers are most common in men aged between 20 and 50 years and in individuals who have type O blood. It is now well recognised that *Helicobacter pylori*, a spiral Gram-negative bacteria, is present in the stomach of over 80% of individuals who present with gastric or duodenal ulcers. The presence of *Helicobacter pylori* leads to impairment of the function of the protective mucosal membrane.

In peptic ulcer disease, erosion of the affected mucosa can lead to haemorrhage, perforation and peritonitis. The typical clinical presentation of duodenal ulcers includes gnawing or burning epigastric pain occurring shortly after meals, heartburn and nocturnal pain. The epigastric pain can be exacerbated by certain foods (i.e. fatty food) but relieved by others (i.e. milk).

Crohn's disease

Crohn's disease is a chronic inflammatory condition, characterised by periods of remission and exacerbation. It can affect any part of the gastrointestinal tract but occurs most commonly in the terminal ileum. Patients with Crohn's disease develop classical symptoms of diarrhoea and abdominal pain, often associated with weight loss. Crohn's disease and ulcerative colitis are often grouped together under the term inflammatory bowel disease (IBD). The presentation and clinical management of these chronic intestinal disorders are examined in Chapter 6.

Coeliac disease

Coeliac disease is a condition which affects the mucosa of the small bowel due to an abnormal reaction to gluten, a protein found in wheat, oats, rye and barley. The presence of gluten causes malabsorption in the proximal small bowel due to atrophy of the villi and a decrease in the activity and amount of enzymes present in the surface epithelium. Injury to the intestinal villi appears to be due to an abnormal immune response to gliadin, a component of gluten. The exact cause of coeliac disease remains unknown but it is thought to result from a combination of genetic predisposition and environmental factors. Although the disease may present at any age, it is most commonly seen between 30 and 40.

Coeliac disease occurs worldwide but is commoner in northern Europe. The prevalence in the UK is 1 in 2000–8000 but reaches 1 in 300 of the population in parts of Ireland (Jewell 2000). Many mild cases are probably undiagnosed and screening studies of asymptomatic populations suggest a prevalence of 1 in 300 throughout northern Europe.

Clinical presentation of coeliac disease

The clinical presentation of coeliac disease is highly variable, depending on the severity and extent of small bowel involvement. Symptoms include recurrent attacks of diarrhoea, steatorrhoea, abdominal distension, flatulence and stomach cramps. Coeliac disease is associated with autoimmune disorders (thyroid disease, insulin-dependent diabetes mellitus, IgA deficiency, Down's syndrome and inflammatory bowel disease). The pathology of coeliac disease also varies considerably; in severe cases the mucosa looks flat with complete loss of surface villi. Histology shows 'subtotal villous atrophy', accompanied by crypt hyperplasia and an accumulation of plasma cells and lymphocytes in the lamina propria. In cases with less severe atrophy the changes are milder and a few patients may show only partial villous with an increase in the intraepithelial lymphocyte count.

Diagnosis of coeliac disease

Diagnosis is usually made by small bowel biopsy showing evidence of villous atrophy. Elevated blood levels of antigliadin and antiendomysium antibodies are detectable in most untreated cases. These antibodies are a valuable 'screening' test in patients with diarrhoea but they are not a substitute for small bowel biopsy and become negative with successful treatment.

Other investigations are usually unnecessary. Barium follow-through X-rays show dilated loops of bowel, coarse or diminished folds and sometimes flocculation of contrast. Sugar tests of intestinal permeability are abnormal and a modest degree of fat malabsorption is usual.

Management of coeliac disease

The management of coeliac disease involves a permanent gluten-free diet, and the vast majority of patients show a marked improvement following dietary change. As gluten is present in wheat, rye, barley and oats this imposes severe dietary restrictions on the patient, which must be fully explained. Rice and potatoes are satisfactory sources of complex carbohydrate.

Initially, frequent dietary counselling is required to make sure the diet is being observed, as the most common reason for failure to improve with dietary treatment is accidental or unrecognised gluten ingestion. In addition to diet, supportive therapy may include iron supplements, vitamin B_{12} and folic acid. In rare cases patients are refractory to standard treatment and require corticosteroids to induce remission.

Ideally, patients should undergo repeat jejunal biopsy after six months of gluten-free diet to ensure that the small bowel lesion has returned to normal, but this may not be necessary in the majority of patients in whom there is a dramatic clinical improvement.

Nursing priorities in coeliac disease relate to the planning and assessment of care which is focused upon nutritional impairment, diarrhoea and associated feelings of anxiety and embarrassment.

Evidence-based guidelines for the management of coeliac disease have been published by the British Society of Gastroenterology (BSG 2002).

Complications of coeliac disease

This condition brings with it an increased risk of malignancy T-cell lymphoma. Patients can develop ulcerative jejuno-ileitis characterised by deep ulcers in the jejunum with malabsorption. Fever, pain, obstruction or perforation may supervene. Metabolic bone disease is common in patients with long-standing, poorly controlled coeliac disease and is a source of considerable morbidity. This complication is less common in patients who adhere strictly to a gluten-free diet.

Malabsorptive disorders of the small intestine

Tropical sprue

As the name suggests, this disease is found in the tropics. Tropical sprue is a chronic, progressive, malabsorptive disorder. It is similar to coeliac disease in that villous atrophy is present but symptoms do not respond to a gluten-free diet. The epidemiological pattern and occasional epidemics suggest that an infective agent or agents may be involved. Although no single bacterium has been isolated, the condition often begins after an acute diarrhoeal illness. Diarrhoea, abdominal distension, anorexia, fatigue and weight loss are the most common symptoms. In visitors to the tropics the onset of severe diarrhoea may be sudden and accompanied by fever. Tropical sprue is treated with broad-spectrum antibiotics as small bowel overgrowth with *E. coli*, enterobacterium and Klebsiella are often seen. Resulting nutritional deficiences may be corrected with folic acid supplements.

Evidence-based guidelines for the management of a variety of malabsorptive disorders have been published by the British Society of Gastroenterology (BSG 2003).

Bacterial overgrowth

The small intestine normally supports a large number of bacterial flora. These are normally kept in check by intestinal peristalsis, the acidity of chyme leaving the stomach, and the secretion of immunoglobulins into the intestinal lumen by mucosal cells. If one or more of these factors is reduced, bacterial overgrowth may result in malabsorption. Diagnosis is by aspiration of the contents of the jejunum, which will reveal increased numbers of both aerobic and anaerobic organisms. If bacterial overgrowth is present, enzymes in the bacteria can inactivate bile acids, leading to fat malabsorption. The gut flora may catabolise ingested proteins, metabolise sugars and bind vitamin B_{12}. Bacterial overgrowth is treated with antibiotics.

Intestinal resection

The long-term effects of small bowel resection depend on the site and amount of intestine resected and vary from trivial to life-threatening. Following ileal resection, vitamin B_{12} and bile salt malabsorption usually develops. Unabsorbed bile salts pass into the colon, stimulating water and electrolyte secretion and resulting in diarrhoea. If hepatic synthesis of new bile salts cannot keep pace with faecal losses, then fat malabsorption occurs. Another consequence is the formation of lithogenic bile and gallstones. Renal calculi, rich in oxalate, develop. Normally, oxalate in the colon is bound to and precipitated by calcium. Unabsorbed bile salts preferentially bind calcium, leaving free oxalate to be absorbed with subsequent development of urinary oxalate calculi.

Patients have urgent watery diarrhoea or mild steatorrhoea. Contrast studies of the small bowel and tests of B_{12} and bile acid absorption are useful investigations. Parenteral vitamin B_{12} supplementation is necessary. Diarrhoea usually responds well to cholestyramine, a resin which binds bile salts in the intestinal lumen. Aluminium hydroxide may also do this in those unable to tolerate cholestyramine.

Bacterial and viral infections

Improved sanitation has led to a decreased prevalence of infectious enterocolitis in the developed world. However, infectious enterocolitis accounts for up to 50% of all deaths before the age of five worldwide, and over 12 000 deaths each day in the children of developing countries. The small bowel may become infected by any of the following types of agents.

Enterotoxigenic bacteria can produce enterotoxins that stimulate the active secretion of electrolytes into the lumen of the small intestine. This results in watery diarrhoea, which is associated with fever. Examples of enterotoxigenic bacteria are *Bacillus cereus*, *Clostridium perfingens* and *Staphylococcus aureus*.

Penetrating bacteria may invade the mucosal lining of the distal small intestine. They often cause extraintestinal disease, sepsis and fever. *Salmonella typhi* is a common example of penetrating invasive bacteria which damage the intestinal mucosa of the distal small bowel. These often produce scant, bloody, mucoid stools, with fever and faecal polymorphnuclear leukocytes. Examples of invasive bacteria that affect the lining of the small intestine are the *Salmonella* species, *Shigella* species, *Escherichia coli*, *Clostridium difficile* and *Vibrio cholerae*.

Viruses, such as rotavirus and adenovirus, may invade the small bowel mucosa, resulting in diarrhoea and malabsorption.

Parasitic diseases of the small intestine

There are a number of parasitic diseases that affect the small intestine, including giardiasis and cryptosporidiosis.

Giardiasis

Giardiasis is caused by the protozoa *Giardia lamblia* and is often associated with ingestion of contaminated food or water. The parasite can present in two forms: cysts and trophozoites. After a cyst has been ingested orally or nasally it matures, and once in the stomach it releases trophozoites. These adhere to the mucosal lining of the proximal small intestine and initiate an inflammatory response. Most adults with giardiasis are asymptomatic, although non-bloody diarrhoea, headaches, nausea and vomiting can result. Diagnosis is by stool culture for the *Giardia* antigen or by small bowel biopsy examination.

Cryptosporidiosis

Cryptosporidiosis is caused by the sporozoa *Cryptosporidium*. The colon and the small intestine are the most common sites for infection, but *Cryptosporidium* has been found in all areas of the digestive and respiratory tracts. Transmission is usually by the faecal–oral route. The severity of the infection ranges from diarrhoeal episodes, which last for up to four weeks in immunocompetent hosts, to death in individuals who are immunocompromised. Before the 1980s very few cases of cryptosporidiosis had been recorded in humans. However, because immunocompromised patients are susceptible to *Cryptosporidium*, the increase in AIDS has caused a noteworthy rise in the number of cases reported.

Miscellaneous disorders of the small intestine

Protein losing enteropathy

This term is used when there is excessive loss of protein into the gut lumen, sufficient to cause hypoproteinaemia. Less than 10% of plasma protein is normally lost from the gastrointestinal tract. Protein-losing enteropathy occurs in many gut disorders but is most common in those where ulceration occurs. In other disorders protein loss results from increased mucosal permeability or obstruction of intestinal lymphatic vessels. Patients present with peripheral oedema and hypoproteinaemia in the presence of normal liver function and without proteinuria. There may also be features of the underlying cause.

Adverse food reactions

Adverse food reactions are common and are subdivided into food intolerance and food allergy, the former being much more common.

Food intolerance

This is adverse reactions to food that are not immune-mediated and result from a wide range of mechanisms. Contaminants in food, preservatives and lactase deficiency may all be involved.

Lactose intolerance
Lactose intolerence may be as a result of lactase deficiency secondary to a disease process, such as coeliac disease or Crohn's disease. It may also result from decreased time of exposure to the intestinal mucosa, such as in short bowel syndrome or dumping syndrome.

Human milk contains around 200 mmol/l of lactose, which is normally digested to glucose and galactose by the brush border enzyme lactase prior to absorption. In most people lactase deficiency is completely asymptomatic. However, some complain of colicky pain, abdominal distension, increased flatus and diarrhoea after ingesting milk or milk products. Irritable bowel syndrome is often suspected but the diagnosis is suggested by clinical improvement on lactose withdrawal. The lactose hydrogen breath test is a useful non-invasive confirmatory test.

Patients with lactose intolerance should avoid milk and milk products, including cheeses and butters. Some sufferers are able to tolerate small amounts of milk without symptoms.

Food allergies

Food allergies are immune-mediated disorders due to antibodies and hypersensitivity reactions. Up to 20% of the population perceive themselves to suffer from food allergy but only 1–2% of adults have genuine food allergies (Heaney 2000). The most common culprits are peanuts, milk, eggs and shellfish.

Clinical manifestations occur immediately on exposure and range from trivial to life-threatening or even fatal anaphylaxis. Allergic gastroenteropathy has features similar to eosinophilic gastroenteritis, while gastrointestinal anaphylaxis consists of nausea, vomiting, diarrhoea and sometimes cardiovascular and respiratory collapse. Fatal reactions to trace amounts of peanuts are well documented.

The diagnosis of food allergy is difficult to prove or refute. Skin prick tests and measurements of antigen-specific IgE antibodies in serum have limited predictive value.

Treatment of proven food allergy consists of detailed patient education and awareness, strict elimination of the offending antigen and in some cases antihistamines. Anaphylaxis should be treated as a medical emergency with resuscitation, airway support and intravenous adrenaline. Subsequently patients should wear an information bracelet and be taught to carry and use a preloaded adrenaline syringe.

Small bowel tumours

Benign or malignant neoplasms of the small bowel make up less than 5% of all gastrointestinal tumours. Small bowel tumours may be primary or secondary carcinomas, carcinoids or lymphomas (Clark *et al.* 2000). Presenting symptoms may include small bowel obstruction, abdominal pain, gastrointestinal bleeding and weight loss. The patient's stools may contain occult blood. Diagnosis is by blood results, barium contrast X-rays, endoscopy and biopsy examination or CT scan.

Benign tumours

The most common benign tumours are adenomas, leiomyomas and lipomas. Adenomas are most often found in the periampullary region and are usually asymptomatic, although occult bleeding or obstruction due to intussusception may occur. Transformation to adenocarcinoma is rare. Multiple adenomas are common in the duodenum of patients with familial adenomatous polyposis (FAP) who require regular endoscopic surveillance.

Primary/secondary carcinomas
Most primary carcinomas of the small bowel are adenocarcinomas and occur in the duodenum. Symptoms include pain, vomiting, anorexia and malaise. Diagnosis is made most commonly by barium X-ray.

Carcinoid tumours
Carcinoid tumours are derived from enterochromaffin cells and are most common in the ileum. Carcinoid tumours also occur in the rectum and in the appendix; the latter are usually benign. Overall, these tumours are less aggressive than carcinomas and their growth is usually slow. Treatment for a carcinoid tumour is by surgical resection. The treatment of patients with carcinoid syndrome is palliative because hepatic metastases have occurred, although prolonged survival is common. Surgical removal of the primary tumour is usually attempted and the hepatic metastases are often excised as reduction of tumour mass improves symptoms.

Lymphomas
Lymphomas of the gastrointestinal tract may be primary, with or without involvement of the adjacent nodes, or secondary, having spread from elsewhere. Non-Hodgkin's lymphoma may involve the gastrointestinal tract as part of more generalised disease or may rarely arise in the gut, with the small intestine being most commonly affected. Lymphomas occur with increased frequency in patients with coeliac disease, AIDS and other immuno-deficiency states. Colicky abdominal pain, obstruction and weight loss are the usual presenting features and perforation is also occasionally seen.

The diagnosis is made by small bowel biopsy, radiological contrast studies and CT scan. Surgical resection, where possible, is the treatment of choice, with radiotherapy and combination chemotherapy reserved for those with advanced disease. The prognosis depends largely on the state at diagnosis, cell type and patient age.

Often metastatic tumours require palliative surgery to relieve obstruction and bleeding. Radiation and chemotherapy of small bowel tumours have been shown to be largely ineffective.

Conclusion

The small intestine receives the contents of the stomach and also, at the duodeum, secretions from the gall bladder and the pancreas. The proximity of the duodenum to the stomach means that this is the prime site for peptic ulcers; the stomach is well protected against the acidity of its contents but the duodenum is less well adapted to this high acidity. The small intestine is the major site of absorption in the gastrointestinal tract and disorders of the small intestine tend to have a deleterious effect on absorption.

One of the first events in the small intestine is the neutralisation of the acid contents of the stomach as they enter the duodenum, by the copious secretion of sodium bicarbonate from the pancreas. Apart from the importance of this process to digestion in the small intestine, which takes place in a neutral to slightly alkaline environment, there is another consequence which can be deleterious to the intestine. Any bacteria, viruses or parasites which have survived the acidic environment of the stomach may have the opportunity to grow in the less hostile environment of the small intestine and this means that the small intestine is the prime site in the gastrointestinal tract for infectious and parasitic diseases. These are all debilitating and, in some cases, life-threatening disorders. The small intestine is also the site where food intolerance and food allergies are manifested.

Nursing care of patients with disorders of the small intestine will involve the usual reinforcement of medical diagnoses. Patients with acute gastrointestinal infections may require intensive care and will require attention to fluid and electrolyte levels as well as nutritional status if they are unable to eat normally. Advice on lifestyle change will be a major feature of nursing care for patients who have intolerant and allergic conditions.

BACKGROUND READING

Additional reading to support the material in this chapter can be found in the relevant sections of the following texts:

Alexander, M., Fawcett, J.N. and Runciman, P. (2000) *Nursing Practice: Hospital and Home – the Adult*. Churchill Livingstone, Edinburgh (Chapter 4).

Brooker, C. and Nicol, M. (2003) *Nursing Adults: the Practice of Caring*. Mosby, London (Chapter 22).

Clancy, J. and McVicar, A.J. (2002) *Physiology and Anatomy: a Homeostatic Approach*, 2nd edition. Arnold, London (Chapter 10).

Clancy, J., McVicar, A.J. and Baird, N. (2002) *Perioperative Practice: Fundamentals of Homeostasis*. Routledge, London (Chapter 2).

Haslett, C., Chilvers, E.R., Boon, N.A. and Colledge, N.R. (2002) *Davidson's Principles and Practice of Medicine*, 19th edition. Churchill Livingstone, Edinburgh (Chapter 17).

Hinchliff, S., Montague, S. and Watson, R. (1996) *Physiology for Nursing Practice*, 2nd edition. Baillière Tindall, London (Chapter 5.1).

Kindlen, S. (2003) *Physiology for Health Care and Nursing*. Churchill Livingstone, Edinburgh (Chapter 9).

Kumar, P. and Clark, M. (2002) *Clinical Medicine*, 4th edition. Saunders, Edinburgh (Chapter 6).

McKenry, L.M. and Salerno, E. (1998) *Pharmacology for Nursing*, 20th edition. Mosby, St Louis (Unit 11).

Watson, R. (2000) *Anatomy and Physiology for Nurses*, 11th edition. Baillière Tindall, London (Chapter 20).

EVIDENCE-BASED GUIDELINES

BSG (2002) *Interim Guidelines for the Management of Patients with Coeliac Disease* (http://www.bsg.org.uk/clinical_prac/guidelines/coeliac.htm accessed 8 May 2004).

BSG (2003) *Guidelines for the Investigation of Chronic Diarrhoea (Tests for Malabsorption)*, 2nd edition (http://www.bsg.org.uk/clinical_prac/guidelines/chronic_diarr.htm accessed 8 May 2004).

REFERENCES

Clark, M.L., Talbot, I.C., Thomas, H.J.W. and Williams, C.B. (2000) Tumours of the gastrointestinal tract. In: *Concise Oxford Textbook of Medicine* (Leadingham, J.G.G. and Worrell, D.A., eds), pp. 577–84. Oxford University Press, Oxford.

Heaney, M.R. (2000) Immune disorders of the gastrointestinal tract. In: *Concise Oxford Textbook of Medicine* (Leadingham, J.G.G. and Worrell, D.A., eds), pp. 591–95. Oxford University Press, Oxford.

Jewell, D.P. (2000) Coeliac disease. In: *Concise Oxford Textbook of Medicine* (Leadingham, J.G.G. and Worrell, D.A., eds), pp. 577–84. Oxford University Press, Oxford.

Misiewicz, J.J. and Punder, R.E. (2000) Peptic ulceration. In: *Concise Oxford Textbook of Medicine* (Leadingham, J.G.G. and Worrell, D.A., eds), pp. 530–37. Oxford University Press, Oxford.

Chapter 6
The Large Intestine

Chapter objectives

After reading this chapter you should be able to:

- Describe the normal anatomy and physiology of the large intestine.
- Understand the physiology of absorption, secretion and motility in the large intestine.
- Identify the range of disorders of the large intestine.
- Relate the pathophysiology, diagnosis and treatment of a number of clinical disorders of the large intestine to nursing care.

ANATOMY AND PHYSIOLOGY

The last 150 cm of the digestive tract are the colon. It is a tube of approximately 4–6 cm in diameter and it extends from the ileo-caecal valve to the anus. The arrangement of the large intestine and its associated structures is shown in Figure 6.1.

The large intestine can be divided up into various regions: the caecum, the ascending colon, the transverse colon, the descending colon, the sigmoid colon and the rectum. The rectum is the portion beyond the sigmoid colon.

Consistent with other regions of the digestive tract, the wall of the large bowel is composed of four distinct layers: the mucosa, the submucosa, the muscularis and the serosa.

In the large intestine the outer longitudinal smooth muscle layer is arranged in three prominent bands, known as taeniea coli. These are shorter than in the small bowel, causing the mucosal lining to pucker and form small sacs called haustra. The size and shape of haustra vary with the state of contraction of the circular and longitudinal muscular layers. These muscular bands are shorter than the longitudinal muscle bands of the colon. Together these two features provide a sacculated appearance to the bowel. Auerbach's plexus is located between the circular and longitudinal muscle layers in the large bowel.

The large bowel has no villi, only the presence of projections. The luminal surface appears much smoother than that of the small bowel. One consequence

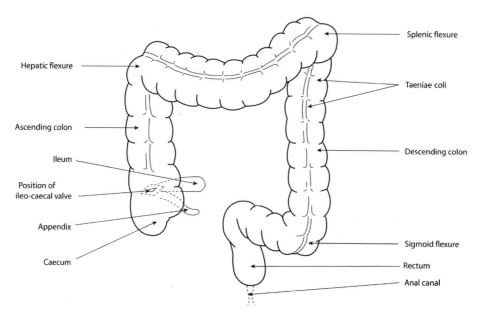

Figure 6.1 Arrangement of the large intestine and its associated structures. Reproduced with permission from Hinchliff *et al.* (1996).

of this structural difference is that the surface area of the large intestine is only one-thirtieth of that in the small intestine.

At the distal end of the ileum, a flap known as the ileo-caecal valve acts as a physiological sphincter both to control the passage of intestinal contents from the small intestine to the large intestine and to prevent any reflux of bacteria from the colon back into the small bowel. The pressure of the ileo-caecal valve is about 20 mm Hg above normal colonic pressure in an average adult.

The caecum forms a blind-ended pouch that is wider in diameter than it is long and which sits below the junction of the small and large intestines. Attached to the end of the caecum is the vermiform appendix. The appendix is a thin, tubular finger-like projection that can range from 5 to 20 cm in length and is about 8 mm in diameter. It has no known digestive role in humans.

Immediately above the caecum is the ascending (right) colon, which passes up the right-hand side of the abdomen to the lower part of the liver, where it bends left at the hepatic flexure (right colic flexure). The transverse colon travels across the abdomen from right to left, from the hepatic flexure to the splenic flexure (left colic flexure). The descending colon runs down the left-hand side of the abdomen from the spleen to the iliac crest, where it forms the sigmoid colon.

The last portion of the large intestine is the rectum. It is about 15 cm long in adults. The distal portion of the rectum forms the anal canal, beginning where the rectum narrows markedly. The surface of the upper anal canal exhibits a number of folds, known as anal (or rectal) folds. Depressions between anal columns are known as anal sinuses. These sinuses end abruptly at the lower end of the columns, in a region known as the dentate line, where there are small crescent-shaped folds of mucosa around the wall. These folds form the anal valve. The anal canal is surrounded by sphincter muscles that control the release of faecal material. The internal anal sphincter is a thickening of the circular layer of the muscularis externa. The external sphincter is composed of skeletal muscle.

The arrangement of the anal sphincters is shown in Figure 6.2.

Blood supply to the large intestine

The right-hand side of the large intestine receives its blood from the branches of the superior mesenteric artery, and the left-hand side and lower portions receive blood from the inferior mesenteric artery. Venous blood from the large bowel is drained mainly through the superior and inferior mesenteric veins.

The rectum and anal canal receive arterial blood from the haemorrhoidal artery, which branches from the inferior mesenteric artery. The rectum also receives arterial blood from branches of the hypogastric artery.

Nerve suppy to the large intestine

The ascending colon, and most of the transverse colon, are innervated by the parasympathetic vagus nerve. The remaining segments receive parasympathetic innervation via branches of the sacral nerves and sympathetic innervation via

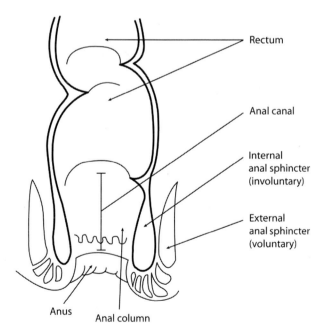

Figure 6.2 Arrangement of the anal sphincters. This material is used by permission of John Wiley & Sons, Inc. From G.J. Tortora *et al. Principles of Anatomy and Physiology*, 8th edition (1996).

the spinal nerves. Stimulation of parasympathetic nerves increases intestinal contraction and the production of mucus. Conversely stimulation of sympathetic nerve fibres inhibits colonic secretions and motility and stimulates the rectal sphincter.

Afferent sensory nerve fibres are present in the mucosa, submucosa and muscular layers of the colon. The colon is insensitive to painful stimuli but is sensitive to changes in pressure. Stretching of the colon as a result of over-distension can result in abdominal pain, but removal of lesions, such as colonic polyps, can be achieved painlessly without anaesthetic.

Functions of the large intestine

The main functions of the large bowel are secretion of a mucinous fluid; the storage and movement of intestinal contents; absorption of water, some electrolytes and bile acids; and excretion of mucus and bicarbonate.

Secretion in the large intestine

The large intestine secretes a thick mucinous secretion, which has a high content of water, mucus, potassium and bicarbonate ions. The alkaline mucus lubricates the intestinal walls, protects the mucosa from acidic bacterial action and helps lubricate the passage of stool.

Secretion in the colon is stimulated by distension and by the mechanical irritation of the colonic walls. Secretomotor neurones from the submucosal and myenteric plexus stimulate secretion through the release of acetylcholine and vasoactive intestinal peptide (VIP). Stimulation of the parasympathetic pelvic nerves also results in secretion. Stimulation of the sympathetic nerves suppresses secretion in the large intestine due to the release of adrenalin and somatostatin. One clinical implication of this is the use of somatostatin analogues in the treatment of secretory diarrhoea.

Motility in the large intestine

The motor function of the large bowel serves both to mix the contents of the lumen and to propel them towards the anus. The chyme enters the colon in a semi-liquid state, but water is absorbed from it and residual matter gradually becomes more solid as it travels through the large bowel. A major function of the rectum is to store faecal material. The passage of food through the stomach and small intestine usually takes less than 12 hours, but a meal residue can remain in the large bowel for a week or more.

There are two basic patterns of movement in the colon:

- Periodic, uncoordinated tonic contractions or segmentations of the circular muscles. This type of segmental motility is known as haustration. The rectum is more active in segmental contraction than the colon.

- Propulsion of chyme towards the anus by segmental propulsion, peristalsis and peristaltic mass movements. Spontaneous movements occur three to four times a day when the colon is full and distended.

When the movements of the sigmoid colon move the faeces into the rectum, the urge to defaecate is stimulated, causing peristaltic waves in the rectum and relaxation of the internal followed by the external anal sphincter. If relaxation of the anal sphincters is not sufficient to allow defaecation, a Valsalva manoeuvre may assist the process. A Valsalva manoeuvre aids the defaecation process by contraction of the diaphragm, thoracic and abdominal muscles.

Control of motility in the large intestine
Motility in the colon is controlled by intrinsic nerves of the intramural plexi and by extrinsic autonomic nerves. Intrinsic nerves, which release acetylcholine, stimulate motility. Extrinsic nerves, which release vasoactive intestinal peptide and nitric oxide, inhibit it. The importance of the intrinsic nerve plexi to the normal functioning of the large intestine is illustrated by the clinical condition Hirshsprung's disease, which is characterised by an absence of intramural ganglion cells in a region of the colon.

Extrinsic autonomic nerves are also involved in the control of the colon. They synapse with neurones in the plexi to modulate the effects of the intrinsic innervation, and innervate colonic smooth muscle directly. Stimulation of the parasympathetic nerves increases motility, whereas stimulation of the sympathetic nerves inhibits motility.

Reflex control of the large intestine

Distension of certain regions of the colon can result in relaxation in other parts. This is known as the colono-colic reflex. Additionally other regions of the digestive tract can reflexly influence colonic motility. The presence of food in the stomach can have a marked influence upon motility in the large intestine; this is known as the gastro-colic reflex and occurs three to four times a day. The gastro-colic reflex is dependent upon the parasympathetic innervation of the colon and the presence of the hormones gastrin and cholecystokinin.

Defaecation

Faeces

In the human adult approximately 150 g of faecal material is eliminated each day. Of this, two-thirds are water and one-third solid. The solid components of faeces comprise undigested cellulose, intestinal bacteria, cell debris, bile pigments and some salts. There is a high content of potassium ions in faeces owing to the secretion of the ions from the colonic walls. The brown colour of faeces is due to the presence of the bile pigment stercobilinogen. The odour is caused by products of protein catabolism and bacterial fermentation in the gut.

Defaecation is a reflex response to the sudden distension of the walls of the rectum. It is a result of mass movements in the colon moving faecal material towards it.

The defaecation reflex has four components:

- increased activity in the sigmoid colon
- distension of the wall of the rectum
- reflex contraction of the rectum
- relaxation and opening of the internal and external anal sphincters.

Control of defaecation is basically an intrinsic reflex mediated by impulses in the internal nerve plexi, which is reinforced by an autonomic reflex transmitted in the spinal cord. However, higher centres are also involved in the regulation of defaecation. When faeces enter the rectum, distension of the wall activates pressure receptors. These send afferent signals through the myenteric plexus to initiate peristaltic waves of muscular contraction in the descending and sigmoid regions of the bowel and the rectum. These waves force faeces towards the anus. As the waves approach the anus, the internal sphincters are inhibited and they relax. The external anal sphincter is innervated by somatic motor nerves and therefore is under voluntary control. If the external sphincter is relaxed voluntarily when the faeces are propelled towards it, defaecation will occur. This is an intrinsic reflex involving parasympathetic nerve fibres in the pelvic nerves, which innervate the terminal colon.

Impact of emotions on defaecation

The effect of emotions upon colonic motility has been studied in several conditions of the large bowel. Patients with irritable bowel syndrome commonly report exacerbation of symptoms at times of emotional stress.

Absorption and digestion in the large intestine

Of the 1000–2000 ml of semi-liquid chyme that enter the colon each day, only 150–200 ml of this material are evacuated in stool. The main reason for this relates to the efficient removal of water in the colon, up to 80–90% from the material that enters the colon.

Electrolytes and water

The absorption of ions and water occurs mainly in the proximal region of the colon. The net absorption of sodium and chloride occurs via exchange mechanisms, similar to the process in the ileum. The neural control of absorption of water and ions is via the enteric nerve plexi. Hormonal control of water absorption in the colon is achieved by production of aldosterone. Anti-diuretic hormone (vasopressin) decreases water absorption in this region.

Intestinal bacteria

Most of the microbial cells that colonise the body reside in the large intestine. A large number of bacteria are excreted in human faeces and more than 99% of these bacteria are non-sporing, anerobes. Apart from these anerobic bacteria, lactobacilli and coliforms also reside in the large bowel. These bacteria synthesise vitamins which are required by the body: vitamins of the B complex (thiamine, riboflavin and vitamin B_{12}) and vitamin K. The production of vitamin K is of particular importance but it is deficient in the average diet and is required for normal blood clotting. Vitamin K is fat-soluble and is therefore easily absorbed in the large bowel. Other vitamins are absorbed by passive diffusion in the colon, and a small number of vitamins which have moved to the small intestine via reflux may be absorbed in this region.

Intestinal bacteria also display digestive functions. They are involved in the conversion of primary bile acids to secondary bile acids and in the deconjugation of conjugated bile acids. Colonic bacteria also convert bilirubins to colourless derivatives known as urobilinogens, which are absorbed directly into the blood. These pigments are mostly excreted in the bile but some are excreted in the urine. Urobilinogen remaining in the gut is partially reoxidised to strercobilinogen, the reddish-brown pigment responsible for the colour of faeces.

PATHOPHYSIOLOGY OF THE LARGE INTESTINE

Among the diseases and disorders that affect the large bowel are intestinal polyps, irritable bowel syndrome, diverticular disease, inflammatory bowel disease and tumours of the colon.

Colonic polyps

Colonic polyps are elevated areas above the mucosal surface into the lumen of the bowel. Polyps range in appearance from tiny translucent and almost invisible bumps only 1–2 mm in diameter to those having a head 1–3 cm in diameter on a vascular stalk. They may be single or may occur together in small numbers, or in hundreds. Diagnosis is achieved by colonoscopy or proctosigmoidoscopy. Most polyps are asymptomatic, but some patients experience intermittent bleeding which can cause mild anaemia. Very large polyps can result in excessive mucus production, altered bowel habit and abdominal pain.

Non-neoplastic polyps make up the vast majority of epithelial polyps found in the large intestine (about 90%); these increase in frequency with age (Clark *et al.* 2000). Endoscopic removal of polyps (polypectomy) greatly reduces the risk of development of cancer.

Colonic diverticulosis

Definitions related to colonic diverticulosis:

- Diverticulum: an outpouching of the wall of the colon.
- Diverticulosis: the presence of diverticula.
- Diverticulitis: more than one diverticula are inflamed.
- Diverticular disease: inflammed diverticula.

Diverticular disease

Diverticular disease is a general term which encompasses diverticulosis and diverticulitis. Diverticular disease has a high prevalence in the Western world, affecting up to 50% of all adults over the age of 70 (Mortensen and Kettlewell 2000). It is characterised by herniation at weak points on the intestinal mucosa and submucosa. A diverticulum typically has a narrow neck that contains all four mucosal layers, and a spherical sac that contains intestinal serosa and mucosa only. Ninety-five per cent of diverticular disease patients have diverticula of the sigmoid colon. Endoscopic presentation of diverticular disease is shown in Plate 6.

Contributing factors for diverticular disease include:

- hypertrophy (enlargement of tissue) of segments of the colon's circular muscle
- age-related atrophy or weakness in the bowel muscles
- increased intracolonic pressure
- chronic constipation and straining
- irregular, uncoordinated bowel contractions
- lack of dietary fibre
- obesity

Possible complications of diverticular disease include ruptured or inflamed diverticulum; abcess formation around the diverticulum; oedema and spasm related to inflammation; erosion of an artery or vein; and colonic fibrosis and narrowing.

Treatment of mildly symptomatic diverticular disease usually involves the diet, most often in the form of a high-fibre diet, and the use of bulk-forming laxatives to help maintain a regular, soft stool. In extreme acute attacks of diverticular disease, bed rest, antibiotics and analgesia may be required.

Diverticulosis

Diverticulosis is uncomplicated diverticular disease. Patients with diverticulosis show no signs of infection; most are asymptomatic. When symptoms are reported, they commonly include diffuse abdominal pain that may be chronic or intermittent and is affected by eating or bowel evacuation, and constipation alternating with diarrhoea. Diagnosis of diverticulosis is confirmed by colonoscopy or barium enema.

Diverticulitis

Diverticulitis is an inflammation in the wall of the diverticulum which occurs most often in the sigmoid colon. Common symptoms of diverticulitis are fever, nausea and vomiting, left lower quadrant abdominal pain and constipation.

Parasitic infections of the large intestine

There are a number of parasitic diseases that affect the large intestine, including amebiasis and trypanosomiasis.

Amebiasis

Amebiasis is a form of colitis caused by the protozoan *Entamoeba histolytica*. It is mainly transmitted by faecal contamination of water or food. Ingested cysts form trophozoites in the small bowel. The amoebae penetrate host tissues causing necrosis without inflammation. Carriers of *Entamoeba histolytica* are often asymptomatic but may suffer from amoebic diarrhoea. Diagnosis of amebiasis requires demonstration of *Entamoeba histolytica* trophozoites and cysts in stool samples. Amebiasis is usually treated with dramatic effect with oral antibiotics, most often diodohydroxyquin.

Trypanosomiasis

Trypanosomiasis is a chronic illness caused by the protozoan Trypanosoma. *Trypanosoma cruzi* causes Chagas' disease, which is transmitted primarily by the reduviid bug's bite but may also be related to blood transfusion or contaminated food. Symptoms of Chagas' disease are anorexia; nausea and vomiting; generalised lymphadenopathy; diarrhoea; cardiac arrhythmias; congestive heart failure; and frequently death. Symptomatic Chagas' disease is largely confined to rural South America. Diagnosis requires identification of *Trypanosoma cruzi* in tissues or blood. Treatment involves prolonged use of antibiotics. Surgery may be required to treat the megacolon (massively enlarged colon).

Further information on parasitic disorders has been written by Francis *et al.* (2003).

Intestinal obstruction

Congenital or acquired intestinal obstructions may occur in either the large or small intestines. The source of obstruction may be neurogenic, vascular or mechanical.

Neurogenic obstruction (intestinal pseudo-obstruction)

In neurogenic obstruction, there is no mechanical blockage of the intestine. Obstruction results from ineffective intestinal peristalsis. Clinical symptoms include pain from intestinal distension, and patients may be cachexic. Diagnosis is made by observation of abdominal distension, gastric aspiration and lack of flatus. Neurogenic obstruction is treated by nasogastric suction and intravenous fluid administration to correct electrolyte imbalances.

Vascular obstruction

A vascular obstruction occurs in the large bowel when an artherosclerotic narrowing interrupts the blood supply to the bowel. This narrowing inhibits peristalsis and can lead to life-threatening intestinal ischaemia in less than one hour. Symptoms include abdominal pain, vomiting, intractable constipation and abdominal distension. Intervention strategies for patients with vascular intestinal obstruction involve the following:

- Regulation of fluids and electrolytes (intravenously).
- Administration of analgesia and anti-emetics.
- Restoration of bowel patency.
- Use of nasogastric suction to relieve abdominal distension.
- Administration of antibiotics to treat bacterial growth.

After abdominal distension has been controlled, surgical intervention may be required depending on the source of the obstruction.

Mechanical obstruction

Mechanical obstructions that are related to congenital defects include stenosis, hernia and aganglionic megacolon (Hirschprung's disease). Hirschprung's disease is a familial disease affecting 1 in 5000 live births (Wright and Walker-Smith 2000). It results from absent intramural ganglion cells in the nerve plexus, most commonly in a segment of the distal colon. As a result the internal anal sphincter fails to relax and constipation and vomiting can develop shortly after birth.

Hirschprung's disease is due to a defect during embryonic development. It is diagnosed by barium enema and anorectal manometry. Treatment involves surgery to remove or counterbalance the obstructing effect of the diseased segment.

Inflammatory bowel disease

Introduction

Crohn's disease and ulcerative colitis are idiopathic chronic diseases. Although they are generally recognised as distinct clinical syndromes they are very closely related illnesses and are commonly grouped together under the term inflammatory bowel disease (IBD). In this section nursing care will be examined without distinction between Crohn's disease and ulcerative colitis. Current best practice in IBD has been published by the BSG (1996).

The prevalence of Crohn's disease varies between geographical locations. It affects 5 in 100 000 of the population in Northern Europe, the United States of America and Australia but appears less common in other areas of the world. It is likely that 20 000–30 000 individuals are affected in the UK (www.bsg.org.uk accessed 8 May 2000).

Crohn's disease occurs more frequently among Caucasians than those of Asian and African origins. The incidence of Crohn's disease in British Asians is higher than in natives from the Indian sub-continent. Similarly, among Afro-Caribbeans the incidence of Crohn's disease is greater in black British West Indians than in native Africans. Crohn's disease is three to eight times more common among Jews than non-Jews and is more common among whites than non-whites.

These findings, however, must be interpreted with caution as access to health care and diagnostic facilities vary between regions and may vary for populations in the same region. Nonetheless they do suggest that a modernised industrialised environment may contain aetiological factors and co-factors for IBD.

The frequency with which Crohn's disease has been diagnosed rose steadily from the 1950s for about 20 years. This may have been due to increased diagnostic awareness as well as a true increase in disease frequency; the disease frequency has stabilised in the last 20 years.

Crohn's disease can present at any age although it most commonly develops between 15 and 30 years of age. It occurs equally commonly in men and women and, at least in the UK, is unaffected by social class.

Ulcerative colitis affects 10 in 100 000 of the general population and is nearly twice as common as Crohn's disease. There are no associations with race, gender and social class. The median age of incidence lies between 15 and 30 years with a second peak between 55 and 70 years, although no age is exempt (www.bsg.org.uk accessed 8 May 2004).

Predisposing factors

There are many suggested predisposing factors related to the development of IBD. The tendency for IBD to occur in populations living in Northern Europe and North America has inevitably suggested a causal link with dietary habits, particularly with dietary fibre and sugar consumption.

Since IBD tends to develop in young adults, factors occurring in childhood have been proposed; breast feeding exerts a protective influence, but whether protection is a direct consequence of breast feeding or whether it arises from associated factors is unknown. One factor may be smoking and there is a large body of evidence indicating that patients with ulcerative colitis are likely to be non-smokers, whereas those with Crohn's disease tend to be smokers. Patients with Crohn's disease who do smoke have more relapses, hospital admissions, surgery and higher blood leukocyte counts than non-smokers. Thus smoking may be a risk factor for the development of Crohn's disease and is associated with more severe disease.

Studies have shown that both Crohn's disease and ulcerative colitis occur more commonly than expected by chance within families. For example, a study in Wales showed that the prevalence of IBD in siblings of patients affected by Crohn's disease was almost 30 times greater than the community prevalence. In addition, when one of the diseases occurs in one family member, the same disease is more likely to manifest itself within the family. This pattern could arise from either common, predisposing genetic factors within the family or common environmental influences.

Aetiology and pathogenesis

Notwithstanding the genetic and environmental predisposing factors, the aetiology of both Crohn's disease and ulcerative colitis remains unknown. It is still debated whether Crohn's disease and ulcerative colitis are separate diseases or whether they represent a continuous spectrum of inflammatory bowel disease.

There is continuing speculation that Crohn's disease may be related in some way to mycobacterial infection, although immunological and therapeutic studies do not show evidence of mycobacterial infection in the majority of cases.

The pathogenesis of the disease is also unclear. The major hypothesis of the pathogenesis of inflammatory bowel disease relates to abnormal immune responses and dysfunctional immune-regulation within the bowel wall. Psychosocial factors related to IBD are addressed in Chapter 13.

Ulcerative colitis

Ulcerative colitis is an inflammatory disorder of the colonic mucosa. The disease is characterised by a chronic relapsing and remitting course. The dominant symptom in ulcerative colitis is diarrhoea, which is usually, but not always, associated with blood and/or mucus in the stool. The endoscopic appearance of ulcerative colitis is shown in Plate 4.

Onset of ulcerative colitis is usually gradual, but it can be abrupt and there may be a previous history of episodic diarrhoea. Loose bowel movements are a consequence of the inflamed rectum, and bowel frequency is related to the severity of the disease. Plate 5 shows an endoscopic view of ulcerative colitis in the rectum.

Abdominal pain is not a prominent symptom for most patients with ulcerative colitis, but mild colicky pain or lower abdominal discomfort relieved by defaecation may be present in some patients. In severe disease, patients can present with fever, weight loss, malaise and lethargy. Weight loss is largely due to diminished food intake secondary to anorexia. Systemic features of anaemia, such as shortness of breath and ankle swelling, may also be present. Extra-intestinal manifestations of ulcerative colitis affect 10–20% of patients; these include primary sclerosing cholangitis, erythema nodosum, pyoderma gangrenosum, iritis and arthritis (Jewell 2000a).

Ulcerative colitis commonly follows a chronic intermittent course, marked by long periods of quiescence interspersed with acute attacks lasting for weeks or months. The reason for these relapses is usually unknown but several causative factors have been postulated, including seasonality, drug ingestion and emotional stress.

Diagnosis is based upon a history of chronic bowel disorder with sigmoidoscopic appearances of granularity, friability and bleeding confirmed by histological examination of rectal biopsies. The extent of the disease is defined by colonoscopy or air contrast barium enema.

Disease severity in ulcerative colitis

Severe ulcerative colitis is defined as the passage of six or more bloody stools daily with systemic disturbances including fever, tachycardia, anaemia or an elevated erythrocyte sedimentation rate (ESR). Mild disease consists of four or less stools per day with little or no blood, the absence of systemic illness or an elevated erythrocyte sedimentation rate. Moderate disease is classified as being intermediate between mild and severe (see Table 6.1).

Complications of ulcerative colitis

Toxic dilatation
Toxic dilatation is defined as dilatation (> 6 cm) of the colon associated with severe, fulminant disease. It is a feature of pan-colitis and most commonly

Table 6.1 Disease severity in ulcerative colitis (Truelove and Witts 1955).

Feature	Mild	Moderate	Severe
Motions a day	< 4	4–6	> 6
Rectal bleeding	Small	Moderate	Large amounts
Temperature	Apyrexial	Intermediate	> 37.8°C
Pulse rate	Normal	Intermediate	> 90 beats a minute
Haemoglobin	> 11 g/dl	Intermediate	< 10.5 g/dl
ESR	< 30 mm/h	Intermediate	> 30 mm/h

occurs at the first presentation of the disease. Features include severe bloody diarrhoea, abdominal pain, pyrexia and tachycardia. Without prompt treatment, toxic dilatation may lead to perforation and generalised peritonitis.

Colonic cancer

Patients with extensive colitis have an increased risk for the development of colonic cancer, although the magnitude of risk is as yet undefined. Prior to the development of cancer, colonic biopsies may show dysplasia, and for this reason screening colonoscopy is undertaken in patients with extensive colitis of more than 10 years' duration.

Massive haemorrhage

Massive haemorrhage may be life-threatening, but is rare. More frequently, bleeding is chronic and insidiously leads to anaemia.

Perianal disease

Although perianal abscess and fistula may develop in ulcerative colitis, they are more common in Crohn's disease.

Medical management of ulcerative colitis

The major medical therapy for active disease is to treat with corticosteroids, such as prednisolone, and when the acute disease has settled, to maintain remission with compounds containing 5-aminosalicylic acid (5-ASA). Azathioprine is used as a 'steroid sparing agent'. Anti-diarrhoea agents, anti-spasmodics, and analgesics are also sometimes used to reduce symptoms without affecting disease activity.

Corticosteroids

Steroids have a wide range of actions in the human body, one of which is a general ability to reduce inflammation. Two steroids in particular, hydrocortisone and prednisolone, have been used with good effect in the management of IBD for many years. Systemic, intravenous steroids are given for very severe or fulminant relapses of ulcerative colitis. Oral steroids are used for slightly less severe exacerbations. Active rectal and sigmoid colitis is treated using corticosteroids in liquid or foam enema preparations. These are relatively convenient to use and have few side-effects. Corticosteroid use is associated with unpleasant side-effects including weight gain, acne, fluid retention and psychiatric symptoms such as mood swings. In the long term they also cause metabolic bone disease and hypertension. It is for these reasons that their use must be closely monitored and limited to acute exacerbations. There is no evidence that they maintain remission, and long-term use of corticosteroids is therefore avoided.

5-Aminosalicylic acid compounds

Only 4% of untreated patients with ulcerative colitis failed to have a further attack of their disease in the 15 years after onset. Maintenance of remission is therefore an important aspect of the long-term management (Jewell 2000a). Over 50 years ago it was noted that the medication, sulphasalazine, used in rheumatological conditions was efficacious in IBD. Sulphasalazine is broken down by colonic bacteria to release an active component, 5-ASA. Consequently, the active drug is only released in the colon. Newer compounds such as osalazine and mesalazine deliver 5-ASA to the colon without the carrier molecule (sulphonamide). Sulphasalazine is one of the mainstays of maintenance therapy in ulcerative colitis. It reduces the frequency of recurrent attacks and is effective over many years. It is also effective in the treatment of mildly active disease.

The reported dose-related side-effects of sulphasalazine include nausea, vomiting, diarrhoea, azospermia and headaches and occur in up to 20% of patients. In cases of sulphasalazine intolerance, hypersensitivity or male infertility the use of mesalazine or olsalazine is indicated. These drugs are appreciably more expensive than sulphasalazine, but are much better tolerated (Jewell 2000a).

Immunosuppressive therapy

Azathioprine and 6-mercaptopurine have been used extensively in IBD. They have been mostly used in Crohn's disease but have also been shown to be effective in the treatment of active ulcerative colitis. They act by damping down immune reactions, probably by indirectly blocking the synthesis of DNA and by direct action on types of white blood cells associated with inflammation. However, their action is slow and they have to be taken for over three months for benefit. Immunosuppresive therapies are particularly helpful in producing remission and preventing relapse in IBD.

The main reluctance to use immunosuppressive drugs is primarily related to their potential toxicity, including bone marrow suppression, hepatotoxicity and acute pancreatitis. Therefore patients must be closely monitored using laboratory tests. Fear concerning their mutogenic and teratogenic potential has been eliminated.

Antibiotic therapy

Antibiotics have long been viewed as a potential treatment option in inflammatory bowel disease in specific clinical situations. Metronidazole is a useful agent for managing peri-anal disease and may also suppress Crohn's disease activity. Other antibiotics have a role in treating septic complications.

Surgical management of ulcerative colitis

The majority of patients with ulcerative colitis can be successfully managed by careful medical management. A minority still require surgical treatment either for fulminating disease, because they are unresponsive or have side-effects from medical treatment, or because quality of life is poor.

Indications for surgery during an acute attack include the presence of a major complication such as perforation or acute dilatation, failure to improve with five days of intensive corticosteroid treatment and reactivation of colitis after the completion of an intravenous corticosteroid regime.

In chronic disease the most common indications are frequent attacks of colitis, not adequately controlled by long-term 5-ASA acid therapy, continuous symptoms in spite of all forms of medical therapy, the development of a complication such as perianal disease or a serious systemic complication such as pyoderma gangrenosum.

Surgery is sometimes indicated to prevent colonic cancer. It is established that patients with ulcerative colitis have a higher incidence of colorectal cancer than the general population and this may be heralded by cytological changes within colonic biopsy specimens (dysplasia).

The standard operative procedure is a total colectomy with an ileostomy. More recently colectomy and formation of an ileo-anal pouch has become the operation of choice for selected patients, since this overcomes the need for a permanent ileostomy.

Crohn's disease

Crohn's disease is characterised by chronic transmural granulomatous inflammation, with a tendency to form complications such as fistulae or strictures. Crohn's disease can affect any area of the gastrointestinal tract, often in discontinuity. The nature and presentation will vary according to the site, the extent of the macroscopic change and presence of complications. Crohn's disease most commonly affects the terminal ileum and proximal colon. Some patients have isolated small bowel or exclusively colonic involvement.

Diagnosis of Crohn's disease

Diagnosis of Crohn's disease, as with ulcerative colitis, is based upon the clinical history of the patient in conjunction with physical findings, laboratory data and endoscopic and radiological examinations. In most patients a good quality barium follow-through or barium enema examination will identify the characteristic features and define the site of macroscopic disease.

Types of Crohn's disease

Colonic disease
The commonest symptoms of extensive colonic involvement are diarrhoea and general malaise, often associated with anorexia and weight loss. Unlike the pattern in small intestinal Crohn's disease, obstructive symptoms are uncommon, though vague persistent abdominal discomfort is often a feature. Left-sided disease is commoner in older patients and symptoms can mimic diverticular disease, with attacks of pain in the left lower abdominal quadrant

and intermittent diarrhoea. Crohn's colitis may be complicated by colonic perforation leading to an acute abdominal emergency.

Perianal disease
Perianal disease is present in more than two-thirds of patients with Crohn's disease, though it is often painless and asymptomatic. Perianal disease only becomes painful when there is local abscess formation or active anal fissure.

Small bowel disease
Ileal disease presents with abdominal pain, diarrhoea and an abdominal mass. Severe symptoms with general malaise, anorexia, weight loss and peripheral oedema, together with a low serum albumin, may occur. Occasionally patients present with fever and right lower quadrant abdominal pain as a result of localised peritonitis.

Gastroduodenal Crohn's disease
Crohn's disease affecting the gastroduodenal region occurs in fewer than 5% of patients and is usually associated with macroscopic disease in other parts of the gastrointestinal tract. Symptoms may resemble that of peptic ulcer disease and include epigastric pain, nausea and postprandial vomiting.

Extra-intestinal manifestations in Crohn's disease

Extra-intestinal manifestations of IBD occur in approximately 15% of all Crohn's disease patients but in up to 30% of those with colonic disease (Jewell 2000b). The extraintestinal features present in Crohn's disease are similar to those experienced in ulcerative colitis. They include erythema nodosum, peripheral arthritis and ocular lesions. Less commonly (< 5%), patients report pyoderma gangrenosum, primary sclerosing cholangitis, renal complications and ankylosing spondylitis.

Some of these manifestations occur during active phases of the disease and respond to treatment of the bowel disorder, others (e.g. ankylosing spondylitis and hepatic complications) appear completely unrelated to disease activity.

Assessment of disease activity in Crohn's disease

Objective scoring of disease activity is important in the assessment of severity of disease and response to treatment. The most commonly used activity assessment tool is the Crohn's Disease Activity Index (CDAI), which is summarised in Table 6.2. Symptoms and physical and laboratory manifestations of Crohn's disease are recorded and assigned a weight. Disease activity is determined from the overall score derived, as shown in Table 6.3. The Harvey–Bradshaw Index and Dutch Activity Index are also widely used in clinical studies (Harvey and Bradshaw 1980). The measurement of health-related quality of life in Crohn's disease is discussed in Chapter 14.

Table 6.2 Crohn's Disease Activity Index.

(x2)	1	Number of liquid or very soft stools in 1 week.
(x5)	2	Sum of 7 daily pain ratings: 0 = none, 1 = mild, 2 = moderate, 3 = severe.
(x7)	3	Sum of daily ratings of general well-being: 0 = generally well, 1 = slightly below par, 2 = poor, 3 = very poor.
(x20)	4	Symptoms or findings presumed related to Crohn's disease: (a) Arthritis/arthralgia (b) Skin/mouth lesions, pyoderma gangrenosa/erythema nodosum (c) Iritis/uveitis (d) Anal fissure, fistula or perirectal abscess (e) Other bowel-related fistula (e.g. enterovesicle) (f) Fever over 37.8°C.
(x30)	5	Use of loperamide or other opiate for diarrhoea: 0 = no, 1 = yes.
(x10)	6	Abdominal mass: 0 = absence; 0.4 = questionable; 1 = present.
(x6)	7	47 minus haematocrit (males); 42 minus haematocrit (females)
(x1)	8	100 × [minus (body weight/standard weight)]

These eight criteria comprise the CDAI. Weighting for each in brackets.

Table 6.3 Disease activity and CDAI score.

	Mild disease	Moderate disease	Severe disease
Score recorded	< 150	150–250	> 250

Complications of Crohn's disease

Oral lesions

Aphthous ulceration is the most common oral complication of Crohn's disease. Ulcers can be extensive and painful enough to impair nutrition. They often occur in association with intestinal disease and respond to treatment directed at the bowel.

Small bowel obstruction

In Crohn's disease small bowel obstruction results from strictures due to fibrosis, with superimposed spasm, inflammation or intestinal adhesions. Patients with Crohn's disease present most commonly with partial small bowel obstructions, which usually respond to medical treatment. Intravenous hydration, nasogastric suction, corticosteroids and parenteral nutrition often lead to prompt resolution of symptoms.

Abscess formation

Abscesses result from either local perforation proximal to a stricture, a penetrating ulcer or inflammatory change in locally involved lymph nodes. This complication leads to pain with anorexia, weight loss, fluctuating fever and general malaise.

Fistulae

The transmural inflammatory nature of Crohn's disease predisposes to the formation of a fistula. The presence of fistulae is usually indicative of active disease and this complication may respond to the medical treatment that is aimed at the Crohn's disease. Enterocutaneous fistulae commonly occur after the incision and drainage of a local abscess and may follow surgery. Spontaneous enterocutaneous fistulae are rare, but can arise in association with recurrent disease.

Entero-enteric fistulae usually occur between adjacent loops of small bowel. They do not usually cause specific symptoms and therefore do not affect clinical management, which is determined by the nature and severity of the underlying disease. Entero-enteric fistulae may occasionally give rise to blind loop syndrome and malabsorption.

Haemorrhage

Massive haemorrhage is a rare but important complication of Crohn's disease. It may occur from ulcers proximal to a tight stricture, owing to erosion of a major artery.

Management of Crohn's disease

The treatment of Crohn's disease encompasses a multi-disciplinary approach including drug therapy, dietary manipulation, replacement of nutritional deficits and surgery. An holistic approach involving psychosocial aspects is important in improving quality of life and this is addressed in detail in this study.

Drug therapy

Drugs used in the treatment of Crohn's disease can be broadly grouped into anti-inflammatory compounds, drugs that may act by affecting immune responses, anti-bacterial drugs and symptomatic treatments.

Anti-inflammatory drugs

Sulphasalazine
Sulphasalazine has been widely used in the medical therapy of Crohn's disease. Unfortunately, sulphasalazine is less than ideal as many patients suffer side-effects (abdominal discomfort, nausea, vomiting and headache). Today there are newer aminosalicylates, particularly Pentasa®, which are released in the ileum as well as the colon and that may have some value in preventing relapse of small bowel disease.

Corticosteroids
The main role of corticosteroids in the medical mangement of Crohn's disease is to suppress acute inflammation of the gut. Currently hydrocortisone,

prednisolone or methylprednisolone are used for severely ill patients in high doses equivalent to 60–80 mg of prednisolone a day. Oral prednisolone in doses of 40–60 mg a day is effective at achieving remission in less severely ill patients. Corticosteroids are of no benefit, however, at maintaining remission in Crohn's disease.

The new steroid preparation, budesonide, is as effective as prednisolone in treating active disease, but because it is then efficiently removed from the circulation by hepatic metabolism it has few steroid-related complications.

Topical corticosteroids available as foams, suppositories and enemas are a useful treatment for inflammation of the distal colon, anal canal and perianal skin.

Combination therapy

It has been demonstrated that remission can be induced more readily by sulphasalazine combined with prednisolone than by sulphasalzine alone. Combination therapy therefore is commonly employed for the induction of remission in Crohn's disease and may be necessary in some cases for the maintenance of remission.

Immunosupressants

Azathioprine and 6-mercaptopurine

6-Mercaptopurine (6-MP) is a purine antagonist, which interferes with nucleic acid synthesis. Azathioprine is largely converted to 6-MP in the body and both drugs have similar clinical effects. Both drugs act slowly over several months and exert a steroid-sparing and anti-inflammatory effect in patients with chronic active Crohn's disease. Azathioprine is used extensively in Crohn's disease patients who have reported side-effects whilst using steroids, or for those who relapse rapidly when steroids are reduced. Azathioprine also appears to have uses in maintaining remission in Crohn's disease. Reluctance to use these drugs is primarily related to their potential toxicity and in one large controlled study about one in ten patients reported that they were unable to take these drugs because of side-effects.

Antibiotic therapy

Antibiotic therapy may reduce secondary infection and reduce the antigenic stimulus of enteric bacteria. Metronidazole has a marked antibacterial action against anaerobic organisms, such as *Clostridium difficile*. Treatment of Crohn's disease with metronidazole as a primary therapy has shown it to be superior to placebo and as effective as sulphasalazine.

Ciprofloxacin is a second antibiotic that, anecdotally, appears to be useful in the treatment of Crohn's disease. Fistulae and perianal symptoms may resolve and it is suggested that ciprofloxacin may function via an immunological mechanism as well as its role as an antibiotic.

Monoclonal antibodies

Antibodies are an important part of the body's defence mechanism. Of great importance in IBD has been the production of monoclonal antibodies to some of the very damaging inflammatory agents (cytokines) that are overproduced and that cause uncontrolled inflammation. In particular, scientists have become interested in the cytokine, tumour necrosis factor alpha (TNFα). Preliminary findings have shown infliximab, a TNFα inhibitor, can be effective in the treatment of Crohn's disease. Although presently restricted to use in severe Crohn's disease, infliximab may provide scope for further treatments in the future.

Nutrition

Malnutrition is a major problem that frequently complicates IBD patients of all ages. Extensive disease, fistula formation and surgical resection can all contribute to inadequate absorption of essential nutrients. Nutrient losses in IBD occur by way of protein exudation from the inflamed gut, iron loss by bleeding and mineral loss through diarrhoea. Other factors potentially contributing to malnutrition include steroid therapy and increased nutritional requirements caused by fever, malabsorption, internal fistulae or inflammatory activity.

General measures of management imply a balanced diet with sufficient calories, including protein, to maintain weight, and adequate vitamins and minerals to sustain healing and correct or prevent deficiencies. Exceptional measures are those necessary to maintain nutrition in an acutely ill patient; normally administered via enteral or parenteral routes, these treatments are widely utilised to control disease activity in IBD.

Total parenteral nutrition (TPN) has been demonstrated to be effective in controlling the disease activity and complications of Crohn's disease. Elemental diets have also been shown to alleviate disease activity in addition to improving nutritional status. Elemental diets are liquid diets that contain all the nutrients that the human body requires. These nutrients come in a digested form to place minimal stress on the digestive system. Elemental diets supply complete nutritional needs whilst resting the digestive system.

The lower cost and reduced risk of complications with elemental diet favour its use over TPN in patients with Crohn's disease. The only circumstances in which TPN therapy is favoured are limited to patients with a very short gut or when there is near complete obstruction. Elemental diet has been found to be less effective in treatment of patients with ulcerative colitis.

The mechanisms by which such nutritional therapies improve disease activity are unclear but may involve the intestinal adaptive response to 'bowel rest', immunologic effects and nutritional factors. Although nutritional therapies are effective as a method of inducing remission in Crohn's disease, relatively little is known about their use for the maintenance of long-term remission. Various diets, including 'low residue' and 'high-fibre low-refined sugar' diets have been employed in IBD without any proven benefits.

Surgical management of Crohn's disease

Eighty per cent of patients with Crohn's disease require at least one operation and some require three or four surgical procedures. It has been reported that between two and four operations are necessary in most patients.

Not all surgical operations for Crohn's disease involve major intestinal resection. Surgical management may be required simply to drain an abscess, assess painful disease under anaesthesia, excise a fistulous track, refashion a stoma or construct a stoma without resecting the bowel. Obstructed bowel may be rectified by stricturoplasty.

Patients with Crohn's disease face a lifetime disorder, which may have metabolic consequences, in which surgical intervention is common. Patients may have to face the prospect of an intestinal stoma and may be worried about the influence of their disease or the effect of surgical treatment on their social, sexual and family lives. These psychosocial issues are given further consideration in Chapter 13. Surgical treatment, however, is an important and established method of treatment. Furthermore, there is no evidence that the role of surgery is diminishing, despite the advances of drug therapy.

Indications for surgery

Surgical interventions for Crohn's disease are usually performed for the complications associated with the disease. The most common indication is obstruction, particularly in the small bowel, but also in the duodenum, colon and rectum. In Crohn's disease abscesses and fistulae are also important indications for surgical intervention. Extensive Crohn's colitis that has failed to respond to medical management is the most common indication for colectomy, and progressive destructive perianal disease may require proctectomy. Less commonly, surgery is required for acute intestinal haemorrhage, perforation of the small or large bowel, acute fulminating colitis, growth retardation in the adolescent patient and malignant change.

Pseudomembranous colitis

Pseudomembranous colitis is defined as an acute inflammation of the mucosa, with the formation of pseudomembranous plaques overlying an area of superficial ulceration. It is also called pseudomembranous enteritis and *clostridium difficile* associated colitis. These conditions are part of the same disease spectrum, which result from disturbance of the normal intestinal lining.

The majority of cases of psuedomembranous colitis involve toxins produced by *clostridium difficile*, which is a Gram-positive, anaerobic bacteria capable of producing many toxic factors. Infection is usually hospital-acquired and becomes established when the normal colonic bacterial flora is disrupted by antibiotic treatment. It should be suspected in patients who develop diarrhoea within six weeks of antibiotic therapy.

Symptoms of psuedomembranous colitis resemble acute ulcerative colitis and range from mild diarrhoea to fulminant colitis, including profuse and watery diarrhoea, abdominal pain and fever. Complications include toxic megacolon, perforation and severe electrolye imbalance.

Management of psuedomembranous colitis

Management usually involves the discontinuation of the offending drug. Supportive therapy with intravenous fluids and bowel rest is often required. Patients with psuedomembranous colitis should be treated with antibiotics. Preventive measures include the responsible use of antibiotics and improved ward hygiene and disinfection policies.

Radiation enteritis

Radiotherapy may have an effect upon the epithelial lining of the intestine. Radiation enteritis occurs during radiotherapy treatment and is characterised by symptoms of nausea, cramp-like pains and altered bowel habit. The extent of injury relates to the size and timing of radiation dosage and can be controlled by using anti-emetics and anti-diarrhoeal agents. Symptoms usually resolve within six weeks of final dose of radiation but some patients can develop chronic radiation enteritis.

Conclusion

Crohn's disease and ulcerative colitis are potentially serious and even life-threatening chronic conditions that have remitting and relapsing natures. The causes of these conditions remain obscure and the search for environmental factors has only made limited progress. Lack of understanding may lead to distress, anxiety, exclusion, loss of self-esteem and impaired health-related quality of life for people with IBD. Further information for sufferers of Crohn's disease is available from Patient UK (http://www.patient.co.uk/showdoc.asp?doc=222 accessed 8 May 2004).

Irritable bowel syndrome

Irritable bowel syndrome (IBS) is one of the most common gastrointestinal disorders in medical practice and can account for approximately 50% of referrals to gastroenterology outpatient clinics. It is estimated that 10–15% of the general population may have IBS, and it affects females more than males (Smith 2003). It is one of a group of clinically diverse conditions known as functional gastrointestinal (GI) disorders. The symptoms of IBS appear to be due to dysfunction of the intestine and are therefore described as functional, as their occurrence cannot be explained by any underlying biochemical or structural abnormality. Other functional disorders of the GI tract include functional abdominal pain, functional abdominal bloating/distension and functional constipation.

Classical IBS is a chronic condition characterised by a range of symptoms including abdominal pain and altered bowel function. Pain may occur anywhere in the abdomen but is most typical in the lower abdomen. Bowel disturbances are classically described as alternating between constipation and diarrhoea, although two-thirds of patients have a predominant pattern of constipation or diarrhoea.

Patients with IBS commonly report a wide variety of non-colonic symptoms such as dyspepsia, backache and gynaecological and urinary symptoms. Tiredness and lethargy are also very common.

Diagnosis of IBS

The symptoms of IBS may be chronic or recurrent and can vary between patients in nature and severity. Diagnosis must be based on the presence of key symptoms and IBS is diagnosed positively on the basis of symptom criteria and the exclusion of organic GI illnesses. Symptom-based diagnostic criteria have been used to define IBS for some time, initially the Manning criteria in the 1970s followed by Rome I criteria in 1992. The most recent criteria are the Rome II guidelines, which are summarised in Box 6.1.

IBS can affect many aspects of an individual's life – work, leisure, travel and relationships – and these effects have a detrimental effect upon the patient's health-related quality of life.

Aetiology of IBS

There is no universal agreement about the aetiology of IBS; it has been speculated that trigger factors could include stress, lifestyle, candida, prolonged use of antibiotics, post-gastroenteritis, emotional trauma or a combination of these factors.

Box 6.1   Rome II criteria for diagnosing IBS.

These criteria state that, within the preceding 12 months there should be at least 12 consecutive weeks of abdominal discomfort or pain that has two of the following three features:

- relieved with defecation; and/or
- onset associated with a change in frequency of stool; and/or
- onset associated with a change in form of stool.

Pathophysiology of IBS

The underlying cause of IBS is poorly understood because there are no objective or biochemical disease markers. Consequently, treatment options are often focused on the relief of specific symptoms. Several proposed mechanisms to explain IBS symptoms include:

- abnormal perception of gastrointestinal events
- altered intestinal motility
- inflammation due to infection
- reduced gastrointestinal compliance

There is clearly a close relationship between the central nervous system and the gut, referred to as the brain/gut axis. Gut function at the end organ level is controlled by a very intricate nerve supply, the enteric nervous system. The nerve fibres of the enteric system that line the gut transmit messages of sensations and pain to higher centres in the brain via the afferent arm of the autonomic nervous system.

Management of IBS

Pharmacological treatments

Despite the development of several new drugs, current pharmacological treatments have limited value in the management of IBS. Pharmacological options tend to focus upon the predominant IBS symptom(s) and generally treatment is empirical; patients may need to receive a number of different agents. Drugs currently recommended by the British Society of Gastroenterology (2000) are summarised in Table 6.4.

Non-pharmacological interventions: psychological

Although it is unlikely that psychological factors cause IBS, they appear to exert a strong influence on some patients with the conditions. Disturbances of mood such as anxiety and depression have also been shown to influence gastrointestinal functional and to occur commonly in IBS patients.

A clear relationship has been established between psychiatric illness, psychosocial morbidity and IBS in patients who seek medical help. Compared

Table 6.4 Drugs for management of IBS.

Symptom	Drug
Abdominal pain	Anti-spasmodics (mebeverine, alverine citrate)
	Tricyclic anti-depressants (amitriptyline)
	5-HT receptor antagonists/agonists (tegaserod)
Diarrhoea	Anti-diarrhoeal (loperamide, codeine, cholestyramine)
Constipation	Dietary fibre

with healthy volunteers, IBS patients have higher scores for anxiety, hostile feelings, sadness, depression and interpersonal sensitivity as well as sleep disturbance. There is, however, some difficulty in interpreting the implications of the co-morbidity between IBS and psychiatric disorders such as anxiety and depression. For example, although anxiety, via the autonomic nervous system, has direct effects upon the gastrointestinal tract and may lead to exacerbation of pain, it is also reasonable to suggest that the symptom of abdominal pain in itself may lead to increased feelings of anxiety. Thus, anxiety may be a cause or a consequence of the symptoms of IBS. Phrases such as, 'I can't stomach that' or 'gut feeling' highlight the very significant role the gut plays as a vehicle of somatic expression. An understanding of the role of psychosocial factors is therefore required to optimise the nursing care of the IBS patient.

Relaxation therapy, biofeedback, cognitive therapy and gut-directed hypnotherapy are examples of psychological therapies in IBS. These therapies are usually provided by clinical psychologists; however it should be recognised that medical and nursing staff can train to provide psychological therapies. At present there are no specific nurse training programmes for psychological therapies to treat IBS patients. It should be recognised that the availability of psychological therapies is limited in the National Health Service. Best practice guidelines for IBS have been published by the BSG (2000).

Colorectal cancer

Colorectal cancer is the second most common type of cancer in adults in the Western world. In the UK the incidence is 60 in 100 000. Colorectal cancer occurs most frequently in persons over the age of 50 (Clark *et al.* 2000). Approximately 95% of intestinal cancers are adenocarcinomas.

Environmental factors account for 80–90% of colorectal cancers. Risk factors include:

- a family history of colonic cancer
- increasing age
- a diet high in fat and carbohydrate and low in fruit and fibre
- ulcerative colitis for more than seven years

Early detection of colorectal cancer is important; patients with carcinoma limited to the bowel wall have a 75% 5-year survival rate, compared to 5% for patients with disseminated disease (Clark *et al.* 2000).

Clinical features of colorectal cancer

Clinical signs and symptoms of colorectal cancer vary depending on the site of the carcinoma. Tumours in the right side of the colon may result in anaemia from occult bleeding, dull abdominal pain, anorexia and weight loss, lethargy and indigestion. In tumours of the left colon, fresh rectal bleeding is common and altered bowel habits, including constipation, difficulty passing stool and abdominal distension are regularly noted.

Clinical investigations

Ideally, colonoscopy is the investigation of choice to detect colorectal cancer. It is more sensitive than barium enema. Endoscopic appearance of a rectal tumour is shown in Plate 7. In addition, lesions can be biopsied and removed during colonoscopy. Examination with rigid sigmoidoscopy will only detect one-third of tumours. Faecal occult blood (FOB) stool testing is widely advocated in individuals over the age of 50 in the USA to increase the number of early cancers detected.

Management of colorectal cancer

Surgery
Treatment of colorectal cancer depends on the stage of the disease. Most patients with colonic cancer require either curative or palliative surgery, such as bowel resection or stoma formation. Surgery will involve the resection of the tumour and associated blood and lymph vessels. In intestinal cancer, patients may require the formation of permanent or temporary colostomy. Formation of a colostomy involves making an outside opening, or stoma, on the abdomen using a section of the colon.

Stoma care
The nurse who has charge of stoma patients has a responsibility for their nursing care in the immediate pre- and post-operative period, to help them adjust to their new situation and to overcome potential psychological problems, such as difficulties with body-image, as well as providing emotional support, encouragement and advice which may be required. Such patients require conscientious stoma nursing care, with priority given to protecting the skin and to controlling odour and faecal drainage.

The growing awareness of this particular field of nursing has seen the development of nurse specialists in stoma care. Stoma nurses work closely with all members of nursing and medical teams to ensure the successful rehabilitation of stoma patients.

Adjuvant therapy
Nearly two-thirds of patients with colorectal cancer have lymph node or disease spread at presentation and are, therefore, beyond cure with surgery alone. Additional interventions include radiation therapy and chemotherapy.

Prevention and screening of colorectal cancer

There is evidence to suggest that in many instances colorectal cancer may be preventable. Primary prevention relates to dietary and lifestyle advice.

Secondary prevention aims to detect and remove tumours at the earliest possible stage. Colonoscopy is the gold standard but is expensive and requires expertise. Flexible sigmoidoscopy is an alternative option. Nurse endoscopists now commonly perform diagnostic flexible sigmoidoscopy. Widespread screening of faecal occult blood (FOB) is an important screening tool.

Best practice guidelines in screening for colorectal cancer have been published by BSG (2002).

Anorectal disorders

Clinical symptoms of anorectal disorders include rectal pain, rectal bleeding and altered bowel function. Causes include haemorrhoids, anorectal abscess, fistula and rectal prolapse.

Haemorrhoids

There are numerous veins in the anal canal; these are longitudinal and thin-walled. The veins can become dilated and convoluted to produce a condition known as haemorrhoids or piles. They may be divided into two main groups, internal and external. Internal haemorrhoids bulge into the rectal lumen above the internal anal sphincter. External haemorrhoids protrude below the external anal sphincter. Symptoms of haemorrhoids include bright red rectal bleeding, iron deficiency anaemia and rectal pain. Diagnosis can be made by visual examination or proctoscopy. Medical interventions for patients with haemorrhoids involve surgical procedures, such as rubber band ligation and haemorrhoidectomy. Haemorrhoids which do not prolapse through the anal sphincter can be treated by local injection.

The role of the nurse involves the provision of dietary advice; a high fibre diet and adequate fluid intake are recommended. Patients may benefit from warm compresses and analgesic ointments.

Following surgical treatment the patient may complain of severe pain and require analgesia. The nurse should monitor the patient for reactionary haemorrhage, recording the rate and volume of the pulse. Frequent observation of anal dressing and pad will detect any bleeding.

Anorectal abscess

Anorectal abscess occurs when infection causes localised accumulation of pus in the tissue spaces around the anorectum. Patients with Crohn's disease are particularly susceptible to abscess formation. The patient with an anorectal abscess presents with throbbing pain in the anorectum, which can increase when seated. Management involves surgical drainage of the abscess followed by treatment with antibiotics and analgesia. One complication of an anorectal abscess is anorectal fistula.

Anorectal fistula

This term describes a hollow, fibrous tract which leads from the anal canal to the perianal skin. The two main types of anorectal fistulas are an intersphincteric fistula and a transsphincteric fistula. The most predominant symptom of an anorectal fistula is a purulent drainage of pus, blood and mucus. Other symptoms include pruritus, pain and odour. The source of a fistula can be detected on sigmoidoscopy and require surgical management.

Rectal prolapse

This condition is likely to result from continual straining to defaecate, or in cases of chronic diarrhoea. Prolapse may also result from overrelaxed anal sphincters or weak pelvic muscles. Symptoms include a protruding rectal mass that is apparent on defaecation, mucus discharge, rectal bleeding and faecal incontinence. Treatment is mainly to remedy the cause of abnormal bowel function and to reduce the prolapse. This condition may be prevented by avoiding constipation and prolonged straining. The nurse should provide dietary advice and encourage adequate intake of fluids. In severe cases injection treatment with sclerosant may be required. Surgery is rarely performed.

Conclusion

The large intestine is the ultimate reservoir for the waste products of digestion and the site of final absorption of water from foodstuffs. Whilst patients may not be aware of the structure and function of their large intestine, they will be aware of its periodic function of defaecation and also as the site of production of gases from the bacterial action on some of the waste products of digestion. While disturbances to other regions of the gastrointestinal tract may not be noticed immediately, disturbances to the defaecatory functions of the large intestine, such as diarrhoea and constipation, will be noticed rapidly and can cause a great deal of suffering and embarrassment. Eating foods which cause the production of excessive gases in the large intestine can lead to feeling bloated and even to discomfort and pain – the usual cause of the 'sore stomach' often reported by children. The large intestine is also sensitive to emotional changes, for instance, the urge to defaecate which accompanies the 'fight or flight' response to stressful stimuli. In addition, there is an increasing public awareness of cancer of the large intestine.

The range of disorders of the large intestine is wide, from localised, but potentially dangerous, changes such as polyps, and age-related but relatively benign conditions such as diverticular disease. However, the large intestine is also the site of the chronic and debilitating conditions called inflammatory bowel disease. These are especially problematic due to the fact that their causes are unknown and the effectiveness of treatments is limited. As such, the inflammatory bowel diseases bring the patient into contact with the health services on a long-term basis – essentially from diagnosis until the end of life – and nursing is of prime importance in providing information and support. The psychosocial aspects of gastrointestinal disorders are the subject of Chapter 13 and more specific aspects of nursing care are covered there.

BACKGROUND READING

Additional reading to support the material in this chapter can be found in the relevant sections of the following texts:

Alexander, M., Fawcett, J.N. and Runciman, P. (2000) *Nursing Practice: Hospital and Home – the Adult.* Churchill Livingstone, Edinburgh (Chapter 4).

Brooker, C. and Nicol, M. (2003) *Nursing Adults: the Practice of Caring.* Mosby, London (Chapter 22).

Clancy, J. and McVicar, A.J. (2002) *Physiology and Anatomy: a Homeostatic Approach,* 2nd edition. Arnold, London (Chapter 10).

Clancy, J., McVicar, A.J. and Baird, N. (2002) *Perioperative Practice: Fundamentals of Homeostasis.* Routledge, London (Chapter 2).

Haslett, C., Chilvers, E.R., Boon, N.A. and Colledge, N.R. (2002) *Davidson's Principles and Practice of Medicine,* 19th edition. Churchill Livingstone, Edinburgh (Chapter 17).

Hinchliff, S., Montague, S. and Watson, R. (1996) *Physiology for Nursing Practice,* 2nd edition. Baillière Tindall, London (Chapter 5.1).

Kindlen, S. (2003) *Physiology for Health Care and Nursing.* Churchill Livingstone, Edinburgh (Chapter 9).

Kumar, P. and Clark, M. (2002) *Clinical Medicine,* 4th edition. Saunders, Edinburgh (Chapter 6).

McKenry, L.M. and Salerno, E. (1998) *Pharmacology for Nursing,* 20th edition. Mosby, St Louis (Unit 11).

Watson, R. (2000) *Anatomy and Physiology for Nurses,* 11th edition. Baillière Tindall, London (Chapter 20).

BEST PRACTICE GUIDELINES

BSG (1996) *Inflammatory Bowel Disease* (http://www.bsg.org.uk/clinical_prac/guidelines/mainibd.htm accessed 8 May 2004).

BSG (2000) *Guidelines for the Management of the Irritable Bowel Syndrome* (http://www.bsg.org.uk/clinical_prac/guidelines/man_ibs.htm accessed 8 May 2004).

BSG (2002) *Guidelines for Colorectal Cancer Screening in High Risk Groups* (http://www.bsg.org.uk/clinical_prac/guidelines/colorectal.htm accessed 8 May 2004).

Francis, J., Barrett, S.P. and Chiodini, P.L. (2003) Best practice guidelines for the examination of specimens for the diagnosis of parasitic infections in routine diagnostic laboratories. *Journal of Clinical Pathology,* **56,** 888–91 (http://jcp.bmjjournals.com/cgi/reprint/56/12/888.pdf accessed 8 May 2004).

REFERENCES

Clark, M.L., Talbot, I.C., Thomas, H.J.W. and Williams, C.B. (2000) Tumours of the gastrointestinal tract. In: *Concise Oxford Textbook of Medicine* (Leadingham, J.G.G. and Worrell, D.A., eds), pp. 577–84. Oxford University Press, Oxford.

Harvey, R.G. and Bradshaw, J.M. (1980) A simple index of Crohn's disease activity. *The Lancet*, **1**, 514.

Jewell, D.P. (2000a) Ulcerative colitis. In: *Concise Oxford Textbook of Medicine* (Leadingham, J.G.G. and Worrell, D.A., eds), pp. 564–8. Oxford University Press, Oxford.

Jewell, D.P. (2000b) Crohn's disease. In: *Concise Oxford Textbook of Medicine* (Leadingham, J.G.G. and Worrell, D.A., eds), pp. 559–63. Oxford University Press, Oxford.

Mortensen, N. and Kettlewell, M.G.W. (2000) Colonic diverticular disease. In: *Concise Oxford Textbook of Medicine* (Leadingham, J.G.G. and Worrell, D.A., eds), pp. 574–5. Oxford University Press, Oxford.

Smith, G.D. (2003) IBS: nursing management and psychological therapies. *Gastrointestinal Nursing*, **1**(7), 24–9.

Truelove, S.C. and Witts, L.J. (1955) Cortisone in ulcerative colitis, final report on therapeutic trial. *British Medical Journal*, **2**, 1041–8.

Wright, V.M. and Walker-Smith, J.A. (2000) Congenital abnormalities of the gastrointestinal tract. In: *Concise Oxford Textbook of Medicine* (Leadingham, J.G.G. and Worrell, D.A., eds), pp. 576–7. Oxford University Press, Oxford.

Chapter 7
The Liver

<hr>

Chapter objectives

After reading this chapter you should be able to:

- Describe the normal anatomy and physiology of the liver.
- Understand the normal physiology of the liver with respect to bile formation, metabolism, vitamin storage, coagulation and detoxification.
- Identify the range of clinical conditions of the liver.
- Relate the corresponding pathophysiology, diagnosis and treatment of the disorders of the liver to nursing practice.

ANATOMY AND PHYSIOLOGY

The liver is the largest gland in the body and is described as a gland due to its secretory function; it produces bile, which is stored in the gall bladder and subsequently released into the duodenum where it has the function of emulsifying fat – breaking it down physically, as opposed to chemically – in order to prepare it for digestion by lipases secreted by the pancreas and the small intestine.

However the liver, which is located in the upper right area of the abdomen (see Figure 7.1), serves many other functions, which are mainly related to its metabolic activity. The liver could also be described as the powerhouse of the body due to its high level of metabolic activity. This metabolic activity involves the breakdown of fat and glucose, the synthesis and storage of glycogen, the breakdown of amino acids to form urea – the means whereby the body gets rid of excess nitrogen – and the synthesis of proteins. In addition, the liver has a crucial role to play in the breakdown of drugs and toxins in the body, often processing them into less active or less harmful substances for subsequent excretion at the kidneys. Clearly, any pathology of the liver has profound consequences for the rest of the body. The high metabolic activity of the liver, whereby adenosine triphosphate (ATP) is synthesised and broken down, also generates heat and, at rest, the liver is primarily the site in the body where heat is generated.

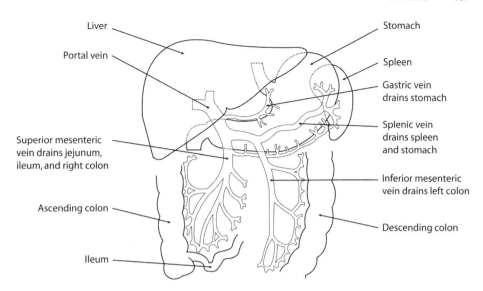

Figure 7.1 Position of the liver in the abdomen. Reproduced with permission from Hinchliff *et al.* (1996).

The liver is composed of highly metabolically active cells called hepatocytes and these are arranged in lobules, with the gross structure of the liver composed of two lobes. Being metabolically active means that the liver requires an adequate supply of oxygenated blood, which is provided by the hepatic artery. Waste substances generated in the liver are removed to the general circulation for excretion by the hepatic vein. However, the liver is unique in having two blood supplies and the second blood supply comes via the hepatic portal veins, which take nutrients from the gastrointestinal tract to the liver.

All of the above – the hepatocytes, the hepatic arterial blood, the hepatic venous blood and the portal blood – are in close proximity in the liver and at a microscopic level in the lobules where arterioles and interlobular veins bring oxygenated blood and nutrients, respectively, from the gastrointestinal tract to the hepatocytes. At the centre of the lobules there is a central interlobular vein, which removes deoxygenated blood and waste products to the venous circulation. Separated from the blood by hepatocytes are the bile canaliculi, which collect bile. Bile is composed of the breakdown products of red cells, which are processed in the liver. Bile is composed of water, bile pigments and bile salts. About a litre of bile is produced daily and this trickles down the bile canaliculi into the hepatic ducts, to the common hepatic duct and into the gall bladder via the cystic duct. The function of the gall bladder is to concentrate bile by the removal of water; this occurs in the presence of fatty foods in the duodenum, which stimulates the release of the hormone cholecystokinin. Cholecystokinin leads to contraction of the gall bladder and the relaxation of the sphincter of Oddi and the release of bile into the duodenum via the ampulla of Vater.

PATHOPHYSIOLOGY OF THE LIVER

The liver is essential to life and has a remarkable capacity to regenerate. Damage to the liver may be acute or chronic. The major causes of liver failure are:

- excessive alcohol
- adverse drug reactions
- viral infections
- biliary obstruction

Pathological conditions which affect the liver are cirrhosis, acute hepatitis, chronic hepatitis and liver tumours.

Cirrhosis

Cirrhosis of the liver is a diffuse and irreversible process associated with progressive liver cell injury and disordered liver architecture. It results in two major events: failure of liver-cell function and portal hypertension.

Cirrhosis is characterised by nodules of hepatocytes separated by intervening fibrosis. It may present as micronodular (nodules of less than 3 mm in diameter), macronodular (nodules of more than 3 mm in diameter) or mixed nodules.

The process of regeneration alters the existing vasculature, resulting in impaired blood flow leading ultimately to hepatic insufficiency.

There are three major aetiological types of cirrhosis.

Alcoholic cirrhosis

Alcoholic cirrhosis is also known as micronodular or portal cirrhosis. It accounts for up to half of all patients. Prognosis in alcoholic cirrhosis depends upon the patient's ability to abstain from alcohol and the degree of hepatic injury at diagnosis.

Primary biliary cirrhosis

Primary biliary cirrhosis and sclerosing cholangitis are immune-related bile duct injuries. These are diseases that predominantly affect middle-aged women. Liver disease in this case is primarily cholestatic, which leads to jaundice, steatorrhea and death from hepatic failure.

Best practice guidelines for the management of biliary cirrhosis have been published by Heathcote (2000).

Postnecrotic cirrhosis

Postnecrotic cirrhosis is caused by hepatic necrosis and can be related to hepatitis, metabolic liver disease and infection. In patients with this type of cirrhosis, the liver can become smaller and distorted.

Physical signs and symptoms of cirrhosis are weight loss, jaundice, anorexia, abdominal pain and bruising. Diagnosis of cirrhosis requires histological confirmation of altered hepatic architecture seen on liver biopsy. The only therapeutic option available for advanced cirrhosis is liver transplantation.

Complications of cirrhosis

Complications of liver cirrhosis include:

- portal hypertension
- oesophageal varices
- ascites
- hepatic encephalopathy

Portal hypertension
When liver blockage leads to increased portal vein resistance and back-flow, portal vein pressure increases. Symptoms of portal hypertension include splenomegaly (enlargement of the spleen), oesophageal varices and haemorrhoids.

Oesophageal varices
Although varices may present in other regions of the digestive tract, they develop most commonly in the submucosal veins of the distal oesophagus and in the stomach. Oesophageal varices are related to portal hypertension, often associated with alcoholic cirrhosis, but may also be seen in patients with chronic hepatitis and portal vein thrombosis. Although the presence of varices may be asymptomatic and variceal bleeding is painless, there is a high risk of rupture in the distal oesophageal veins, which causes potentially life-threatening bleeding. In an acute variceal bleed the patient vomits bright red blood and can develop signs and symptoms of hypovolaemia. Upper endoscopy is used to diagnose, evaluate and treat oesophageal varices (see Chapter 10).

Gastric varices
Portal hypertension may lead to the development of collateral circulation with the formation of varices that carry blood away from the portal circulation. Oesophageal varices are the most clinically significant type; however, many patients with oesophageal varices also have gastric varices. Patients who bleed from gastric varices appear to rebleed and have a high mortality rate. A complete upper endoscopy is required to diagnose variceal bleeding.

Best practice guidelines for the management of variceal bleeding have been published by BSG (2000).

Ascites
Ascites (an abnormal collection of serous fluid in the peritoneal cavity) may be due to intravascular pressure in the capillaries of the liver or hypoproteinaemia. The nurse can partly control the formation of ascites in the cirrhotic patient by reduction in dietary fluid and sodium, bed rest and through the administration of diuretics.

Hepatic encephalopathy
Hepatic encephalopathy is related to large amounts of ammonia within brain tissue. Ammonia is normally produced by the breakdown of protein in the bowel; this is metabolised by the healthy individual to produce urea. In patients with portal hypertension, the blood cannot pass through the liver and the ammonia therefore heads into the general circulation and flows to the brain. Hepatic encephalopathy is classified as a neuropsychiatric complication of liver disease and the main symptoms are confusion and irrational behaviour. It is treated by rectifying the patient's pH and electrolyte levels, restricting dietary protein and preventing gastrointestinal bleeding.

Hepatitis

Hepatitis is defined as an inflammation of the liver accompanied by liver damage. It can be due to infections, usually viral (hepatitis A and B), or damage by drugs or alcohol. Hepatitis can be acute or chronic.

The most prevalent type of hepatitis is viral hepatitis. It may be caused by hepatitis virus A, B, C, D, E or G. Hepatitis may also result from alcohol abuse, it may be drug-induced or may result from autoimmune disease.

Common forms of hepatitis:

- hepatitis A (infectious hepatitis)
- hepatitis B (serum hepatitis)
- hepatitis C (parenterally transmitted)
- hepatitis D

Hepatitis A

Hepatitis A virus is the most common type of hepatitis (Williamson 2003). It is generally a mild disease and is spread by the faecal oral route, either through oral anal sexual practices or by contaminated food or water. Hepatitis A usually presents sub-clinically. Symptoms when present include low-grade fever, fatigue, nausea and malaise, followed by dark urine and light stools. Physical findings include jaundice and tender hepatomegaly (enlarged liver).

Hepatitis B

Hepatitis B virus is a DNA virus that is transmitted via contaminated blood, semen and saliva. Infection with hepatitis B may lead to a chronic liver state, liver cancer or cirrhosis. Fortunately, protection against hepatitis B is available in the form of immunisation.

In uncomplicated cases of hepatitis B, presentation of jaundice and hepatomegaly is accompanied by several symptoms including dark urine, pale stools, lethargy and nausea. Hepatitis B is diagnosed by the presence of hepatitis B surface antibody in blood serum. The vast majority (95%) of individuals who acquire hepatitis B infection recover uneventfully. Treatment involves rest from strenuous activity, nutritionally balanced diet, electrolyte management and, if required, subcutaneous vitamin K can be administered. Patients should be strongly advised to avoid alcohol. Complications of hepatitis B infection include chronic hepatitis, which develops in 10% of patients, and in the most severe cases fulminant hepatic failure, which is usually fatal (Williamson 2003).

Chronic hepatitis

Chronic hepatitis is defined as hepatic inflammation continuing without improvement for longer than six months. A prolonged period of lethargy, jaundice and fluid retention, in conjunction with laboratory findings such as low serum albumin, high gamma globulin and a prolonged prothrombin time, support a diagnosis of chronic hepatitis.

Fulminant hepatic failure

Fulminant hepatic failure is defined as massive liver cell death following the development of acute hepatitis. Patients with fulminant disease are confused and have ascites, oedema, coagulation problems and a shrinking liver. There is a high (> 80%) mortality rate and the only treatment is liver transplantation.

Hepatitis C

Hepatitis C is associated with extrahepatic disease. It may be transmitted parenterally, from mother to baby or through sexual contact. In the Western world most infection is associated with high-risk activities such as intravenous drug use and multiple blood transfusions. The incubation period for hepatitis C is 6–8 weeks and infection is asymptomatic in over 90% of cases. Complications of hepatitis C include chronic hepatitis, cirrhosis and liver cancer.

Best practice guidelines for the management of hepatitis C have been published by BSG (2001).

Hepatitis D

Hepatitis D is caused by a defective RNA virus. It is found worldwide and in the Western world is closely associated with high-risk activity (intravenous drug use). Transmission is usually parenteral.

Alcoholic hepatitis

This is inflammation of the liver caused by alcohol ingestion. Liver biopsy in patients with a history of alcohol abuse demonstrates liver cell degeneration, necrosis and fatty deposits. Symptoms of alcoholic hepatitis include right upper quadrant abdominal pain, fever, vomiting, anorexia and dark urine. Alcoholic hepatitis does not usually present with jaundice. Physical signs include hepatomegaly (enlarged liver), spenomegaly (enlarged spleen) and signs of cirrhosis. Treatment is based upon support care and abstinence from alcohol.

Drug-induced hepatitis

The liver plays a central role in the metabolism and excretion of drugs. At least 10% of all adverse reactions to drugs affect the liver. These reactions can range from asymptomatic to fulminant hepatic failure. Drugs can cause damage to hepatocytes, which is indistinguishable from viral hepatitis and cholestatsis. The mechanism of drug-induced damage includes direct toxicity to hepatocytes, the conversion of a drug into toxic metabolite and a drug-induced autoimmune reaction.

Diagnosis of drug-induced hepatitis is made on the basis of a careful drug history, clinical signs and improvement if the patient stops the offending drug.

Liver tumours

Benign and malignant tumours may arise in the liver from the hepatocytes, bile duct epithelium or supporting hepatic tissue. With the exception of hepatocellular carcinoma, primary malignant tumours of the liver are rare, but the liver is frequently the site of metastatic tumours from other areas in the body (lungs, breast and bronchus). Predisposing factors for primary cancerous liver tumours include a history of cirrhosis, hepatitis B, hepatitis C, alcohol abuse and exposure to hepatotoxic chemicals.

Most patients with liver cancer are asymptomatic until the disease is well advanced. Presenting complaints include:

- right upper quadrant pain
- weight loss
- general lethargy

Physical signs include an enlarged and tender liver. Diagnosis is made by liver biopsy, ultrasound and CT scans.

Treatment of liver tumours

Much of the treatment for hepatic tumours is of necessity only palliative due to the advanced stage of the primary lesion when metastases are present.

Guidelines for the management of liver cancer have been published by BSG (2003).

Conclusion

The liver is one of the vital organs of the body, and while we are generally unaware of its function we are very soon aware of any dysfunction. Its importance as a synthetic and storage organ, in addition to its prime importance in producing body heat, is evident through its regenerative capacity. However, some infections and the abuse of some substances, principally alcohol, cannot be sustained indefinitely and ultimately liver failure will ensue. Cancer in the liver is often secondary to cancer elsewhere in the body and the liver's copious blood supplies (peripheral and portal circulations) and functional proximity to the lymphatic system mean that it is a prime site for metastases. These are invariably fatal.

A patient with liver failure will feel very ill indeed and, due to poor prognosis from liver failure, will be very distressed. The patient may also be disfigured by jaundice, which can be quite frank and alarming in extreme liver failure, and by ascites. In addition to the palliative measures which can be administered to patients with liver failure, a significant aspect of care will involve psychosocial support of the patient and family, and nurses have a major role to play in this regard.

BACKGROUND READING

Additional reading to support the material in this chapter can be found in the relevant sections of the following texts:

Alexander, M., Fawcett, J.N. and Runciman, P. (2000) *Nursing Practice: Hospital and Home – the Adult*. Churchill Livingstone, Edinburgh (Chapter 4).

Brooker, C. and Nicol, M. (2003) *Nursing Adults: The Practice of Caring*. Mosby, London (Chapter 23).

Clancy, J. and McVicar, A.J. (2002) *Physiology and Anatomy: a Homeostatic Approach*, 2nd edition. Arnold, London (Chapter 10).

Haslett, C., Chilvers, E.R., Boon, N.A. and Colledge, N.R. (2002) *Davidson's Principles and Practice of Medicine*, 19th edition. Churchill Livingstone, Edinburgh (Chapter 18).

Higgins, C. (2000) *Understanding Laboratory Investigations: a Text for Nurses and Healthcare Professionals*. Blackwell Publishing, Oxford (Chapter 10).

Hinchliff, S., Montague, S. and Watson, R. (1996) *Physiology for Nursing Practice*, 2nd edition. Baillière Tindall, London (Chapter 5.2).

Kindlen, S. (2003) *Physiology for Health Care and Nursing*. Churchill Livingstone, Edinburgh (Chapter 10).

Kumar, P. and Clark, M. (2002) *Clinical Medicine*, 4th edition. Saunders, Edinburgh (Chapter 7).

McKenry, L.M. and Salerno, E. (1998) *Pharmacology for Nursing*, 20th edition. Mosby, St Louis.

Watson, R. (2000) *Anatomy and Physiology for Nurses*, 11th edition. Baillière Tindall, London (Chapter 21).

BEST PRACTICE GUIDELINES

BSG (2000) *UK Guidelines on the Management of Variceal Haemorrhage in Cirrhotic Patients* (http://www.bsg.org.uk/clinical_prac/guidelines/man_variceal.htm accessed 8 May 2004).

BSG (2001) *Clinical Guidelines on the Management of Hepatitis C* (http://www.bsg.org.uk/clinical_prac/guidelines/hep_c.htm accessed 8 May 2004).

BSG (2003) *Guidelines for the Diagnosis and Treatment of Hepatocellular Carcinoma (HCC) in Adults* (http://www.bsg.org.uk/clinical_prac/guidelines/hcc.htm accessed 8 May 2004).

Heathcote, E.J. (2000) Management of primary biliary cirrhosis. The American Association for the Study of Liver Diseases practice guidelines. *Hepatology*, **31**, 1005–13.

REFERENCES

Williamson, L. (2003) Nursing patients with hepatic, biliary and pancreatic disorders. In: *Nursing Adults* (Brooker, C. and Nicol, M., eds), pp. 621–51. Mosby, London.

Chapter 8
The Biliary System

Chapter objectives

After reading this chapter you should be able to:

- Describe the normal anatomy and physiology of the biliary system, including the gall bladder and its associated duct system.
- Understand the motility and secretory functions of the gall bladder.
- Identify a range of clinical conditions of the biliary system.
- Relate the pathophysiology, diagnosis, and treatment options of biliary conditions to nursing practice.

ANATOMY AND PHYSIOLOGY

The biliary system consists of the gall bladder and its associated duct system – the hepatic, cystic and common bile ducts.

Gall bladder

The gall bladder is a pear-shaped sac. In the human adult it is approximately 8 cm long and 4 cm wide, but is capable of considerable distension. The gall bladder is lined by a mucous membrane, which is thrown into many folds (or rugae) when the gall bladder contracts. When distended the gall bladder has a capacity of up to 50 ml.

The gall bladder is attached to the undersurface of the liver by connective tissue, the peritoneum and blood vessels (see Figure 8.1). The four anatomical divisions of the gall bladder are:

- a distal blind sac, or fundus
- a funnel-shaped body, which connects the fundus to the infundibulum
- the infundibulum, which connects the body to the neck
- the neck

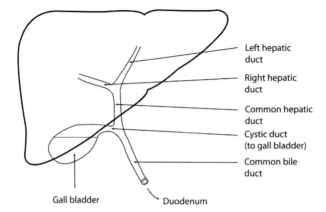

Figure 8.1 Attachment of the gall bladder to the liver. Reproduced with permission from Hinchliff *et al.* (1996).

The wall of the gall bladder is composed of three distinct layers: the mucous membrane, the muscularis and the serosa. The epithelium of the mucous membrane is composed of high columnar cells with basally located nuclei. Around the mucous membrane is a thin coat of smooth muscle, the mucularis externa. Most of the smooth muscle runs obliquely but some runs circularly and some longitudinally. Outside the muscle layer is an outer coat of fibroconnective tissue, the serosa, which is covered by the peritoneum.

At the neck of the gall bladder the mucous membrane is thrown into a spiral fold, which is composed mainly of smooth muscle. This tissue extends into the cystic duct and is known as the spiral valve. It is thought the spiral valve has a role in preventing sudden filling or emptying of the gall bladder.

Blood supply to the biliary system is via the hepatic artery. Venous blood is drained through the cystic vein.

Functions of the gall bladder

The functions of the gall bladder are to store and concentrate bile, and to deliver it to the duodenum during a meal.

Motility

As it emerges from the gall bladder, the cystic duct combines with the common hepatic duct to form the common bile duct, which joins with the main pancreatic duct to form the ampulla of Vater.

During their passage through the duodenal wall, the common bile duct, the pancreatic duct and the ampulla of Vater are surrounded by an arrangement of smooth muscles, the spincter of Oddi. The closure of this sphincter prevents bile from entering the duodenum. This closure results in formed bile being diverted into the gall bladder. The main stimulus for the relaxation of the sphincter muscle is cholecystokinin (CCK). Thus when levels of CCK increase in the blood during a meal, the gall bladder contracts, the sphincter of Oddi

Table 8.1 Electrolytes and organic molecules in gall bladder bile.

Constituent	Bile (mM)
Electrolytes	
Bicarbonate (HCO_3^-)	10
Chloride (Cl^-)	25
Potassium (K^+)	12
Sodium (Na^+)	130
Calcium (Ca^{+2})	
Organic molecules	
Bilirubin	5.1
Cholesterol	16.0
Lecithin	3.9
Bile salts	145.0

relaxes and bile flows into the duodenum. Other factors, such as pharmaceutical agents, sensory input, disease and emotional states, may also influence the filling and contraction of the gall bladder.

Secretion
Bile is an alkaline, greenish-yellow fluid that is secreted continuously by the liver. It is composed of different secretions, one originating in the liver cells (hepatocytes) and the other in the cells which line the bile ducts. The two secretions mix together in the ducts.

Gall bladder bile is an isotonic solution but some of its components are highly concentrated. Its major components are water (which makes up 97% of hepatic bile), bile salts, fatty acids, lipids, inorganic electrolytes and other organic substances (see Table 8.1). When bile flows from the liver through the cystic duct and into the gall bladder for storage, up to 90% of the water is removed.

Bile has a number of functions, which include the emulsification of undigested fats; the activation of both intestinal and pancreatic enzymes; the facilitation of the absorption of fat-soluble vitamins; and providing a route of excretion for bilirubin, cholesterol, thyroid and adrenal hormones. Bile also aids the neutralisation of gastric acid in the small intestine in that its composition is similar to pancreatic juice.

The volume of alkaline secretion, unlike hepatic bile, is not directly determined by the concentration of bile salts in the blood.

Gall bladder contraction
The gall bladder exhibits muscle tone even in the interdigestive period. It also contracts between meals to deliver bile intermittently into the duodenum. The major stimulus for gall bladder contraction after a meal is high blood levels of cholecystokinin (CCK), the duodenal hormone that is released in reponse to fats in the duodenum. Gastrin, which is released in the stomach

antrum in response to peptides in the food, also stimulates gall bladder contraction.

Vasoactive inhibitory peptide (VIP), pancreatic polypeptide and stimulation of the sympathetic nerves to the gall bladder, all cause gall bladder relaxation. Bile acids, by means of feedback control, also inhibit gall bladder contraction.

Bile pigments in the gastrointestinal tract

After delivery to the intestines most conjugated bilirubin is excreted in the faeces. This is due to the intestinal mucosa not being very permeable to the conjugated bile pigment. However, some bilirubin may be deconjugated by the action of bacteria in the intestines and the free bilirubin formed can be partially absorbed. Intestinal bacteria can also convert bilirubin to colourless derivatives known as urobilinogens, which can be absorbed into the portal blood. These are then secreted in bile and urine. Urobilinogen remaining in the intestines is partially reoxidised to stercobilinogen, the reddish-brown pigment responsible for the colour of faeces.

Jaundice

Failure of the body to excrete bile pigments results in accumulation of pigments in the blood plasma, termed hyperbilirubinaemia. This can result from a disruption of the flow of bile through the common bile duct or hepatic ducts by obstruction, i.e. gallstones, allowing bile to build up in the blood.

Bile pigments, mainly bilirubin, are deposited in the skin, mucous membranes and sclera, causing a yellow discoloration commonly known as jaundice. Jaundice is usually persistent and accompanied by severe pruritus (itching). The itching can be all over the body and the patient can scratch until their skin bleeds. Nurses should make every effort to relieve the itching; antihistamines are commonly prescribed but these can cause sedation. Effective relief can be achieved with the use of calamine lotion.

Jaundice is obvious when the plasma bilirubin concentration exceeds 34 μmols/litre. Jaundice can result from excessive breakdown of red blood cells (haemolysis) and haemoglobin to release bilirubin. Consequently the liver's capacity to excrete is overwhelmed; this is known as prehepatic or haemolytic jaundice. The bilirubin present in the plasma in this form of jaundice is largely unconjugated as it has not been taken up and conjugated by the liver.

Other common causes of jaundice include decreased uptake of bilirubin into hepatocytes, defective intracellular coagulation, or disturbed secretion into the bile canaliculi. Jaundice is most often seen in acute hepatitis and is known as intracellular or hepatocellular jaundice.

Gallstones can block the intrahepatic and extrahepatic bile ducts. This can result in jaundice as the bile is refluxed into the blood. This type of jaundice is referred to as obstructive or posthepatic jaundice.

PATHOPHYSIOLOGY OF THE GALL BLADDER

Gall bladder diseases can either be short-term and easily manageable or longer-term and debilitating. Generally diseases of the biliary system present during middle age. In individuals aged 20–50, diseases of the biliary tract are six times more common in women than in men, but over the age of 50 the incidence in men and women becomes equal (Summerfield 2000).

Biliary tract disorders that are examined in this section include cholelithiasis, cholecystitis, choledocholithiasis, cholangitis and carcinoma.

Gallstones (cholelithiasis)

Gallstones are the presence of stones or calculi in the gall bladder. There are two types of gallstone: cholesterol stones and pigment stones. Cholesterol stones make up three-quarters of all gallstones. To understand the mechanisms of gallstone formation it is important to know their composition.

Cholesterol stones

Cholesterol stones contain cholesterol, calcium salts, bile acids, fatty acids, proteins and phospholipids. If the concentration of bile acids or phospholipids drops, cholesterol will not be held in micelles. This results in the bile becoming supersaturated with cholesterol. When the cholesterol is not soluble in this supersaturated system, it forms microcrystals. These microcrystals grow and cluster with one another and with other bile constituents to form gallstones.

Cholesterol gallstones are more prone to develop when there is a high ratio of cholesterol to bile acids or lecithin in the bile. This can be due to high cholesterol levels related to a high fat diet. Gallstones also form when there is a reduction in bile acid secretion, as a consequence of bile acid malabsorption or reduced lecithin secretion.

Risk factors for the formation of both cholesterol and pigment stones are shown in Table 8.2.

Table 8.2 Risk factors for formation of gallstones.

Cholesterol gallstones	Pigment gallstones
Increasing age	Increasing age
Female sex	Chronic haemolysis
Pregnancy/use of oral contraceptive	Alcohol abuse/cirrhosis
Obesity	Biliary infection
Gall bladder staisis	Total parenteral nutrition
Spinal cord injury	Gall bladder stasis

Pigment stones

Pigment stones are far less common than cholesterol stones. They are usually small, only a few millimetres in diameter, and are either dark brown or black. When they occur they are usually multiple. They contain between 40% and 90% pigment and less than 20% cholesterol. Pigment stones account for between 20% and 25% of all gallstones.

Acute cholecystitis

This occurs when gallstones irritate the mucous membrane of the gall bladder, which then becomes inflammed. The patient usually presents with an acute illness, which is severe in nature. The patient may be in shock due to pain and vomiting. The nurse may also notice pyrexia and tachycardia, due to infection. Treatment, cholecystectomy (surgical removal of the gall bladder), is often performed laprascopically, with good effect. The benefits of laprascopic surgery include:

- reduced hospital stay
- minor surgical wound
- earlier mobilisation
- reduced risk of surgical complications
- reduced need for opioid analgesia
- quick return to normal lifestyle

If gallstones are only present in the common bile duct they can be removed via endoscopic retrograde cholangiopancreatography (ERCP). The nursing priorities of care before surgery in acute cholecystitis include:

- Pain control (intramuscular opiate analgesia at regular intervals).
- Hourly monitoring of patient's vital signs until they become stable.
- Fasting the patient and commencing intravenous fluids.
- Intravenous administration of a broad-spectrum antibiotic.
- In the presence of vomiting, a naso-gastric tube may be passed and an antiemetic given.
- Careful monitoring of electrolyte and fluid balance.

Best practice guidelines for the management of acute cholecystitis related to acute pancreatitis have been produced by Glazer and Mann (1998).

Choledocholithiasis

The presence of stones in the common bile duct or hepatic duct is called choledocholithiasis. This condition arises when stones passed out of the gall bladder become lodged in the common bile duct or hepatic duct and prevent the flow of bile into the duodenum. Patients may be asymptomatic or can present with biliary colic, right upper quadrant abdominal pain, obstructive jaundice, acute gallstone pancreatitis and cholangitis. Therapeutic ERCP is the preferred method of medical treatment.

Cholangitis

Cholangitis is a bacterial infection of the bile duct that is associated with obstruction of the common bile duct. Infection may lead to widespread inflammation, which can develop into fibrosis and stenosis of the bile duct. Patients with mild cholangitis report fever spikes, chills, dark urine and abdominal pain. In more severe presentation cholangitis can be devastating, with toxic sepsis, shock and mental impairment. Prognosis in severe cholangitis is poor.

Primary sclerosing cholangitis

Primary sclerosing cholangitis is an inflammatory process that results in multiple strictures of bile ducts, which lead to chronic cholestatic liver disease. The cause of primary sclerosing cholangitis is unknown. However, up to 75% of patients with primary sclerosing cholangitis have ulcerative colitis. Clinical presentation includes fatigue, pruritis (itch), jaundice and abnormal liver function tests (see Chapter 7). Diagnosis is by ERCP and liver biopsy examination. Asymptomatic primary sclerosing cholangitis requires no treatment.

Carcinoma of the biliary tract

Gall bladder cancer

Cancer of the biliary tract usually involves the gall bladder. Gall bladder cancer is usually an adenocarcinoma and occurs far more frequently in women than men. Symptoms usually involve:

- right upper quadrant abdominal pain
- nausea and vomiting
- substantial weight loss
- anorexia

Approximately 80% of gall bladder tumours also have gallstones. Diagnosis is made by ERCP, ultrasound, cholecystogram or cholangiogram. The great majority of these cases can only be treated palliatively (Summerfield 2000).

Carcinoma of the extrahepatic biliary ducts

Tumours of the biliary ducts are extremely rare, usually associated with long-standing primary sclerosing cholangitis. Adenocarcinoma is the most common form of cancer in the biliary tree. Often the patient presents with painless obstructive jaundice. Other features of biliary cancer include:

- substantial weight loss
- pyrexia
- pruritis
- nausea and vomiting

Patients with established biliary cancer rarely survive more than a few months, and treatment is usually palliative. Even with surgical resection and radiotherapy, prognosis is extremely poor.

Conclusion

The biliary system is intimately related in terms of structure and function to the liver and shares a common entrance to the gastrointestinal tract at the duodenum. The biliary system merely concentrates and stores a liver product: bile. While important in fat breakdown, bile is not essential for life. On the other hand, disorders of the biliary system can cause considerable suffering and also disfigurement in the form of jaundice, if the outflow of bile from the gall bladder is blocked.

The structure and function of the biliary system is relatively easy to understand and in turn to explain to patients who may be puzzled at the sudden onset of extreme pain, as in the case of obstruction or inflammation of the gall bladder. The concept of referred pain is also important in any explanation of symptoms to patients. In extreme cases, patients will also wonder why and how they can survive without a gall bladder if it has to be surgically removed. In all of the above, nurses can play a key role in offering information and support to patients with disorders of the biliary system. Likewise, while jaundice can be very distressing and uncomfortable for patients, they can be reassured, in the absence of any liver pathology, that the situation can be resolved effectively.

BACKGROUND READING

Additional reading to support the material in this chapter can be found in the relevant sections of the following texts:

Alexander, M., Fawcett, J.N. and Runciman, P. (2000) *Nursing Practice: Hospital and Home – the Adult.* Churchill Livingstone, Edinburgh (Chapter 4).

Brooker, C. and Nicol, M. (2003) *Nursing Adults: the Practice of Caring*. Mosby, London (Chapter 23).

Clancy, J. and McVicar, A.J. (2002) *Physiology and Anatomy: a Homeostatic Approach*, 2nd edition. Arnold, London (Chapter 10).

Clancy, J., McVicar, A.J. and Baird, N. (2002) *Perioperative Practice: Fundamentals of Homeostasis*. Routledge, London (Section 2).

Haslett, C., Chilvers, E.R., Boon, N.A. and Colledge, N.R. (2002) *Davidson's Principles and Practice of Medicine*, 19th edition. Churchill Livingstone, Edinburgh (Chapter 18).

Higgins, C. (2000) *Understanding Laboratory Investigations: a Text for Nurses and Healthcare Professionals*. Blackwell Publishing, Oxford (Chapter 10).

Hinchliff, S., Montague, S. and Watson, R. (1996) *Physiology for Nursing Practice*, 2nd edition. Baillière Tindall, London (Chapter 5.2).

Kindlen, S. (2003) *Physiology for Health Care and Nursing*. Churchill Livingstone, Edinburgh (Chapter 9).

Kumar, P. and Clark, M. (2002) *Clinical Medicine*, 4th edition. Saunder, Edinburgh (Chapter 7).

McKenry, L.M. and Salerno, E. (1998) *Pharmacology for Nursing*, 20th edition. Mosby, St Louis (Chapter 40).

Watson, R. (2000) *Anatomy and Physiology for Nurses*, 11th edition. Baillière Tindall, London (Chapter 21).

BEST PRACTICE GUIDELINES

Glazer, G. and Mann, M.V. (1998) United Kingdom guidelines for the management of acute pancreatitis. *Gut*, **42**, S1–S13.

REFERENCES

Summerfield, J.A. (2000) Diseases of the gallbladder and biliary tree. In: *Concise Oxford Textbook of Medicine* (Leadingham, J.G.C. and Worrell, D.A., eds), pp. 609–13. Oxford University Press, Oxford.

Chapter 9
The Pancreas

Chapter objectives

After reading this chapter you should be able to:

- Describe the normal anatomy and physiology of the pancreas.
- Understand the normal physiological functions of the pancreas, including both endocrine and exocrine secretions.
- Identify the range of clinical conditions specific to the exocrine function of the pancreas.
- Relate the corresponding pathophysiology, diagnosis and treatment of disorders of the pancreas to nursing practice.

ANATOMY AND PHYSIOLOGY

The pancreas is both an endocrine and an exocrine gland. It is a wedge-shaped elongated gland which lies in the abdominal cavity. It is approximately 15 cm long and 5 cm wide and it weighs about 80–90 g. Structurally the pancreas can be divided into three regions: the head, which lies over the vena cava in the C-shaped curve of the duodenum; the body, which lies behind the duodenum; and the tail, which is situated under the spleen (see Figure 9.1).

The pancreatic duct (duct of Wirsung) runs the whole length of the pancreas from left to right and joins the common bile duct. Pancreatic juice empties from this duct into the duodenum via the ampulla of Vater.

The pancreas is composed of two types of cell, exocrine and endocrine cells.

Exocrine tissue

Pyramidal acinar cells are exocrine cells that compose the bulk of pancreatic tissue. Groups of acinar cells form an acinus, and groups of acini form grape-like lobules. The acini secrete the digestive enzymes of the pancreatic juice. The nucleus of the acinar cell is situated at the base of the cell. The cytoplasm in the basal region can be stained with a dye to show the presence of rough endoplasmic reticulum, the site of digestive enzyme production. Small mito-

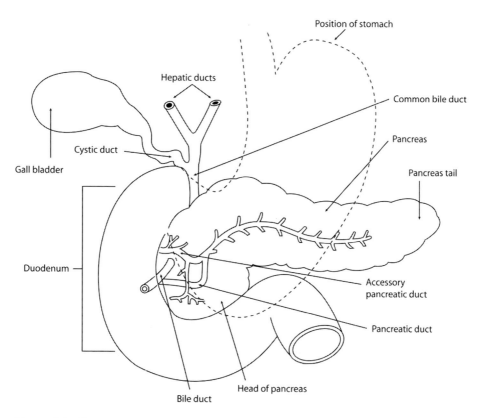

Figure 9.1   Structure of the pancreas. Reproduced with permission from Hinchliff *et al.* (1996).

chondria are situated throughout the acinar cell, and the apical portion of the cell contains the Golgi body, and numerous zymogen granules, which contain the pancreatic enzymes and enzyme precursors.

Each exocrine unit of the pancreas consists of a terminal acinar portion and a duct. The duct that drains from the acinus is known as an intercalated duct, which empties into larger intralobular ducts. The intralobular ducts in each lobule of the pancreas drain into larger extralobular ducts, which empty the secretions of the pancreas into the main collecting duct, the pancreatic duct (see Figure 9.2).

Small mucous glands situated within the connective tissue surrounding the pancreatic duct secrete mucus directly into the duct.

The exocrine units of the pancreas surround the islets of Langerhan, the endocrine units of the pancreas.

Endocrine pancreas

Endocrine cells, or the islets of Langerhan, make up 1% of the pancreatic cells. They are most numerous in the tail region of the pancreas. They consist of

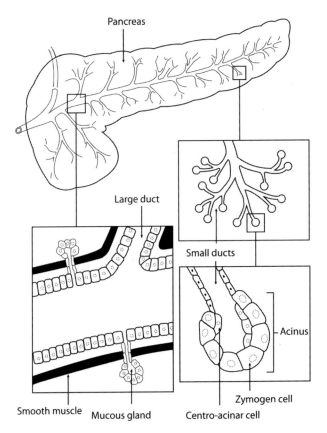

Figure 9.2 Ducts of the pancreas. Reproduced with permission from Churchill Livingstone. From S. Rutishauser, *Physiology and Anatomy: A Basis for Nursing and Health Care* (1994).

clusters of cells surrounded by pancreatic acini and vary in size. As with all endocrine tissue, the hormones they produce are secreted directly into the blood. The major endocrine cells of the pancreas are alpha, beta and delta cells, which secrete glucagons, insulin and somatostatin, respectively. Glucagon (alpha cells) and insulin (beta cells) are taken up by the local blood vessels to act systemically.

When the blood sugar level falls below normal levels, the alpha cells are stimulated to secrete glucagon, which accelerates the conversion of glycogen to glucose in the liver. When the blood sugar level is above normal, the beta cells secrete insulin, which promotes both the metabolism of glucose by tissue cells and the conversion of glucose to glycogen, which is then stored in the liver.

Somatostatin (produced in the delta cells) acts locally in a paracrine manner to inhibit the secretions of alpha and beta cells.

Blood supply to the pancreas

Oxygenated blood is supplied to the pancreas by the branches of the coeliac, splenic and superior mesenteric arteries. The acini and ducts are surrounded by separate capillary beds. Blood drains from the pancreas via the portal vein to the liver or into the splenic circulation by the superior mesenteric and splenic veins.

Nerve supply to the pancreas

Cholinergic preganglionic fibres of the vagus nerve enter the pancreas. They synapse with postganglionic cholinergic nerve fibres, which lie in pancreatic tissue and innervate both acinar and islet cells. Post-ganglionic sympathetic nerves from the coeliac and superior mesenteric plexi innervate vascular flow and control pain sensations and enzyme secretion in the pancreas. Parasympathetic fibres control exocrine and endocrine functions.

Pancreatic juice

The exocrine acinar cells secrete between 500 and 1000 ml of pancreatic juice each day. Pancreatic juice has two types of secretion, an enzyme-rich portion and an aqueous alkaline-rich portion. It is a colourless fluid and has a pH of 8.1–8.3. It consists of water, bicarbonate, sodium, potassium, chloride and calcium. The function of the alkaline nature of pancreatic juice, together with other alkaline secretions, namely bile and intestinal juice, is to neutralise the acidic chyme arriving from the stomach.

This neutralising function is important for three main reasons:

- Pancreatic enzymes require a neutral or slightly alkaline environment for optimal activity.
- The absorption of fat depends upon the formation of micelles in the intestinal lumen, a process which will only take place at a neutral or slightly alkaline pH.
- It protects the intestinal mucosa because excess acid in the duodenum can damage the mucosa and lead to ulceration.

Pancreatic juice enters the duodenum with secretions of the biliary system at the ampulla of Vater.

Pancreatic enzymes

There are three main types of enzyme present in pancreatic juice:

- Amylases, which break down carbohydrates into glucose and maltose.
- Lipases, which are important in the early stages of fat breakdown.
- Proteases, including trypsinogen, the precursor of proteolytic trypsin.

These enzymes are released from the pancreatic acinar cells and are involved in the digestion of foodstuffs. The acinar cells contain zymogen granules, in which enzyme or enzyme precursor proteins are stored. The enzyme precursors produced by the acinar cells include those of the proteolytic enzymes, trypsin and chymotrypsin. The release of enzymes as inactive precursors ensures that the activated enzymes do not autodigest the lining of pancreatic tissue.

Control of pancreatic juice secretion

The control of exocrine secretion of the acinar cells of the pancreas is via peptides, such as the hormones secretin and cholecystokinin, and somatostatin, which acts mainly as a paracrine factor, and via neurotransmitters.

Hormonal control
The main hormones involved in stimulating secretion of pancreatic juice are secretin, which stimulates the secretion of the alkaline aqueous component, and cholecystokinin (CCK), which stimulates the secretion of the enzyme component. These hormones are produced in the duodenal mucosa in response to food constituents in duodenal chyme. As the secretion of pancreatic juice is under the control of two separate regulatory mechanisms, the composition of the juice can vary with regard to its enzyme protein content.

Somatostatin, which is present in the delta cells in the islets of Langerhan of the pancreas, is a powerful inhibitor of pancreatic secretion. It acts in a paracrine manner to inhibit the release of the exocrine alkaline and enzyme secretions, as well as the pancreatic hormones insulin and glucagons. In addition, somatostatin inhibits the release of a number of gastrointestinal hormones, including CCK, secretin and gastrin.

Neural control
The nervous control of pancreatic secretions is via both sympathetic and parasympathetic nerves. Stimulation of cholinergic fibres in the vagus nerve enhances the rate of both alkaline and enzyme fluid. Stimulation of sympathetic nerves inhibits secretion owing to vasoconstriction of blood vessels in the gland, which leads to a decreased volume of juice secreted. At rest, the pancreas secretes enzymes at about 15% of the maximal rate and alkaline juice at less than 2%.

The control of secretion of pancreatic juice during a meal depends upon the volume and composition of the food ingested. Pancreatic secretions occur in the following three phases.

Cephalic phase
The sight or smell of food, or other sensory stimuli associated with the impending arrival of food, elicits increased pancreatic secretion via a conditioned reflex. The presence of food in the mouth stimulates secretion via a non-conditioned

reflex. The control during this phase is therefore nervous and is mediated by impulses in cholinergic fibres in the vagus nerve. This results in a modest output of enzyme-rich pancreatic juice, containing very little bicarbonate.

Gastric phase

The presence of food in the stomach stimulates the secretion of pancreatic juice via a hormonal mechanism. Activation of chemical receptors in the walls of the stomach causes the release of gastrin from G-cells into the local circulation. Distension of mechanoreceptors in the stomach also stimulates secretion. This phase results in a moderate production of pancreatic juice that is rich in enzymes but low in bicarbonate.

Intestinal phase

The intestinal phase is probably the most important phase in response to food. Food material in the duodenum stimulates both the alkaline and enzyme-rich components of pancreatic juice. The alkaline component of pancreatic juice is secreted in response to the presence of acid in the duodenum. Acid also stimulates the release of secretin from cells in the intestine and this hormone stimulates duct cells in the pancreas to secrete alkaline fluid. The enzyme-rich juice released during the intestinal phase is in response to fats and peptides in food. These cause the release of CCK from the walls of the duodenum into the bloodstream. CCK stimulates acinar cells to secrete enzymes. Trypsin in the duodenum inhibits the release of enzymes via the inhibition of CCK; this is a feedback control mechanism which limits the quantity of enzymes in the small intestine and may have a protective function.

In the absence of pancreatic enzymes, up to 35% of dietary fat and protein may be assimilated using less efficient pathways of digestion, such as salivary amylase and the enzymes for the brush border of the gut mucosa. It is estimated that pancreatic enzyme must fall below 10% of normal before maldigestion or malabsorption occurs.

PATHOPHYSIOLOGY OF THE EXOCRINE PANCREAS

Disorders of the exocrine function of the pancreas are an important cause of malabsorption because of the central role of the pancreas in the digestion of fat and protein. Conditions that affect the pancreas include acute and chronic pancreatitis, pancreatic fistulas and neoplasms of the pancreas.

Pancreatitis

Pancreatitis is inflammation of the pancreas that generally results from the obstruction of the pancreatic duct. Pancreatitis may be acute or chronic.

Acute pancreatitis

Acute pancreatitis is a medical emergency, resulting in auto-digestion of the pancreas. It is most commonly caused by excessive alcohol abuse, abdominal trauma, trauma during endoscopic retrograde cholangiopancreatography (ERCP) and bile duct stones. Inappropriate activation of digestive enzymes in the pancreas can result in destruction of the organ with potentially catastrophic consequences. Symptoms of acute pancreatitis include:

- severe upper abdominal pain, which can radiate into the back
- nausea and vomiting
- abdomen tender to palpation
- hypovolaemia and hypotension
- elevated serum amylase and urine amylase

There is no specific test for acute pancreatitis. Diagnosis is usually made by measurement of serum amylase, which is normally greatly elevated in acute pancreatitis. Other diagnostic procedures include ERCP and endoscopic ultrasonography.

The key to treatment of acute pancreatitis is prompt and rapid intravenous fluid replacement aimed at haemodynamic stabilisation, correction of metabolic abnormalities and resting the pancreas. Patients with impaired islet cell function receive insulin to control diabetes.

Best practice guidelines, as outlined above, for the management of acute pancreatitis have been produced by BSG (1998) and by Toouli *et al.* (2002).

Nursing management of the patient with acute pancreatitis involves the following:

- Ensuring adequate pain relief.
- Withdrawal of all food and fluids and nasogastric suctioning to rest the digestive system.
- Bed rest and temperature-controlling measures to reduce metabolic rate to a minimum, which will reduce the secretion of pancreatic enzymes.
- Intravenous electrolyte and fluid replacement.
- Provision of enzyme and vitamin supplements.
- In severe cases, peritoneal lavage may be required.
- Supporting the patient in maintaining personal hygiene.
- Monitoring blood sugar levels in order to detect secondary diabetes.

Investigative procedures for pancreatic disease are often extensive and surgery in the majority of cases only offers palliation. The gastrointestinal nurse has an important role to play in helping both the patient and relatives deal with this difficult time.

The nursing care of patients with acute pancreatitis will vary according to the severity of the attack. Acute pancreatitis is usually treated conservatively as an operation would increase mortality. Complications of acute pancreatitis include infection, respiratory distress, pseudocyst, abscess or pancreatic fistula formation.

Chronic pancreatitis

Chronic pancreatitis is related to acute pancreatitis, usually caused by excessive long-standing alcohol abuse. In chronic pancreatitis the destruction of the pancreas is a slow and progressive disorder (Toskes 2000). It is seen most commonly in male patients aged between 40 and 60 who normally present with:

- prolonged ill-health (abdominal pain, vomiting and nausea)
- weight loss and malabsorption
- steatorrhea (a condition where faeces have a high fat content)
- diabetes mellitus (as a result of islet cell destruction)

The destruction of pancreatic tissue results in secondary calcification in the organ and cystic changes due to obstruction of drainage of the small ducts in the gland. Blood and pancreatic function tests are used to confirm a diagnosis of chronic pancreatitis. ERCP may be used to determine the extent of disease.

Successful management of chronic pancreatitis largely relies on the patient abstaining from alcohol, and on pain relief, nutritional support and oral replacement of digestive enzymes.

Pancreatic pseudocysts

Pseudocysts are localised collections of pancreatic secretions and are a complication of both acute and chronic pancreatitis. They may be single or multiple and are 5–10 cm in diameter. Pseudocysts may produce abdominal pain and, more rarely, haemorrhage, infection and peritonitis. Abdominal ultrasonography, endoscopic ultrasonography and CT scan are the best methods of identifying a pseudocyst or pancreatic abscess.

Pancreatic fistula

Pancreatic fistula may follow trauma to the gland or occur as a complication following pancreatic surgery. The management of pancreatic fistula requires both a nursing and medical management, as the release of pancreatic enzymes onto the skin will quickly cause excoriation. The skin may be protected by the application of barrier creams. Fluid loss and electrolyte balance need to be corrected, either by oral or intravenous route, and drainage from deep in the wound may be carried out by insertion of a drain. About 75% of pancreatic fistulas close spontaneously within six months. If a fistula should fail to close it may require surgical intervention.

Pancreatic cancer

Tumours, wherever they present, are classified as benign or malignant. In the pancreas most tumours are malignant and most commonly affect the exocrine portion of the pancreas. Over 90% of malignant tumours are adenocarcinomas. Pancreatic cancer most often develops in persons aged between 60 and 80. Potential risk factors for the development of a pancreatic tumour include chronic pancreatitis, smoking and a high fat diet. Of pancreatic carcinomas, over 60% occur in the head of the pancreas, 15–25% in the body and 5% in the tail (Russell 2000). Symptoms are most common in tumours of the head of pancreas and typically result in dull abdominal pain, weight loss and obstructive jaundice. Obstruction and/or metastasis may also cause signs and symptom of liver damage (dark urine and light stools). ERCP is the most efficient test for detection of pancreatic cancer. The prognosis for pancreatic cancer is very poor; median survival time is only 2–3 months following diagnosis (Russell 2000). Therefore therapy in pancreatic cancer is primarily palliative and supportive. Most patients present with metastatic disease and are not suitable for curative surgery. The nurse should aim to help the patient reduce the impact of associated symptoms by ensuring pain control and relief from nausea and vomiting.

Surgery for pancreatic cancer

The majority of patients with pancreatic cancer have disease in the head or the neck of the gland. The only curative surgical procedure is a pancreaticoduodenectomy, also known as a Whipple's procedure. In this operation the pancreatic head, neck and body are resected, along with the distal biliary tree and gall bladder. Outcomes in managing pancreatic cancer surgically have improved recently; if surgery is performed before nodal spread takes place, survival rates increase.

Conclusion

Sharing a common route of entry for secretions to the duodenum with the biliary system, the pancreas is intimately anatomically located to several organs including the stomach, liver and spleen. The pancreas has both exocrine activities and endocrine activities as it produces digestive secretions and hormones, which control carbohydrate metabolism. Disorders of the pancreas are serious, usually resulting in both acute and chronic pancreatitis. It is the digestive nature of the organ which leads to problems as the proteolytic enzymes, which it contains, come into contact with surrounding tissues. The intimate anatomical association with several other organs can lead to damage to these organs as well as to the pancreas. Good nursing care is required in terms of pain relief and managing shock in patients with pancreatitis, in addition to support of patients who may have cancer of the pancreas or who may have been abusing alcohol.

BACKGROUND READING

Additional reading to support the material in this chapter can be found in the relevant sections of the following texts:

Alexander, M., Fawcett, J.N. and Runciman, P. (2000) *Nursing Practice: Hospital and Home – the Adult*. Churchill Livingstone, Edinburgh (Chapter 4).

Brooker, C. and Nicol, M. (2003) *Nursing Adults: the Practice of Caring*. Mosby, London (Chapter 23).

Clancy, J. and McVicar, A.J. (2002) *Physiology and Anatomy: a Homeostatic Approach*, 2nd edition. Arnold, London (Chapter 10).

Haslett, C., Chilvers, E.R., Boon, N.A. and Colledge, N.R. (2002) *Davidson's Principles and Practice of Medicine*, 19th edition. Churchill Livingstone, Edinburgh (Chapter 18).

Higgins, C. (2000) *Understanding Laboratory Investigations: a Text for Nurses and Healthcare Professionals*. Blackwell Publishing, Oxford (Chapter 11).

Hinchliff, S., Montague, S. and Watson, R. (1996) *Physiology for Nursing Practice*, 2nd edition. Baillière Tindall, London (Chapter 5.2).

Kindlen, S. (2003) *Physiology for Health Care and Nursing*. Churchill Livingstone, Edinburgh (Chapter 9).

Kumar, P. and Clark, M. (2002) *Clinical Medicine*, 4th edition. Saunders, Edinburgh (Chapter 7).

McKenry, L.M. and Salerno, E. (1998) *Pharmacology for Nursing*, 20th edition. Mosby, St Louis (Chapter 40).

Watson, R. (2000) *Anatomy and Physiology for Nurses*, 11th edition. Baillière Tindall, London (Chapter 21).

BEST PRACTICE GUIDELINES

BSG (1998) *United Kingdom Guidelines for the Management of Acute Pancreatitis* (http://www.bsg.org.uk/clinical_prac/guidelines/acute_pan.htm accessed 8 May 2004).

Toouli, J., Brooke-Smith, M., Bassi, C., Carr-Locke, D., Telford, J., Freeny, P., Imrie, C. and Tandon, R. (2002) Guidelines for the management of acute pancreatitis. *Journal of Gastroenterology and Hepatology*, **17**, S15–S39.

REFERENCES

Russell, R.C.G. (2000) Tumours of the pancreas. In: *Concise Oxford Textbook of Medicine* (Leadingham, J.G.G. and Worrell, D.A., eds), pp. 606–8. Oxford University Press, Oxford.

Toskes, P.P. (2000) Chronic pancreatitis. In: *Concise Oxford Textbook of Medicine* (Leadingham, J.G.G. and Worrell, D.A., eds), pp. 603–6. Oxford University Press, Oxford.

Section 2
Essential Aspects of Gastroenterology

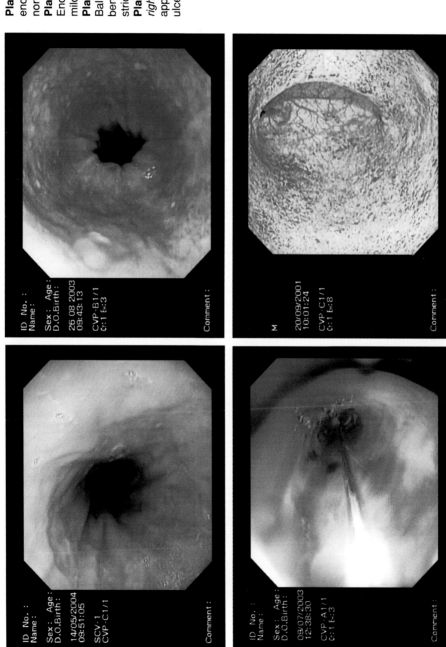

Plate 1 (*top left*) An endoscopic view of a normal oesophagus. **Plate 2** (*top right*) Endoscopic view of mild oesophagitis. **Plate 3** (*bottom left*) Balloon dilation of a benign oesophageal stricture. **Plate 4** (*bottom right*) Endoscopic appearance of ulcerative colitis.

ID No. :
Name :

Sex : Age :
D.O.Birth :

14/05/2004
09:51:05

SCV-1
CVP-C1/1

Comment :

ID No. :
Name :

Sex : Age :
D.O.Birth :

26 08 2003
09:43:13

CVP-B1/1
C:1 E:3

Comment :

ID No. :
Name :

Sex : Age :
D.O.Birth :

09/07/2003
12:38:30

CVP-A1/1
C:1 E:3

Comment :

M

20/09/2001
10:01:24

CVP-C1/1
C:1 E:8

Comment :

Plate 5 (*top left*) Endoscopic appearance of rectal ulcerative colitis.
Plate 6 (*top right*) Endoscopic presentation of diverticular disease.
Plate 7 (*bottom left*) Endoscopic appearance of a rectal tumour.

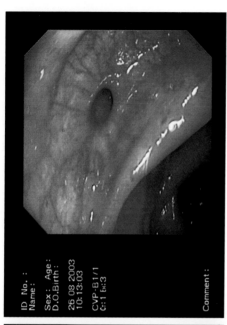

ID No.:
Name:

Sex: Age:
D.O.Birth:

26.08.2003
10:13:03

CVP-B1/1
Gr:1 Ex:3

Comment:

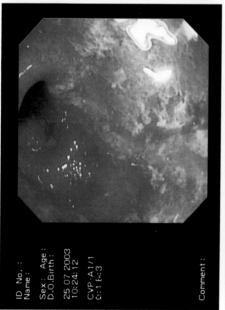

ID No.:
Name:

Sex: Age:
D.O.Birth:

25.07.2003
10:24:12

CVP-A1/1
Gr:1 Ex:3

Comment:

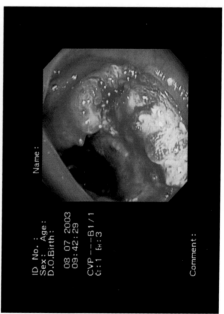

ID No.:
Sex: Age:
D.O.Birth:

Name:

08.07.2003
09:42:29

CVP----B1/1
Gr:1 Ex:3

Comment:

Chapter 10
Diagnostic Procedures and Tests in Gastroenterology

The material in this chapter is presented in two sections: the first considers endoscopy and the second considers a range of tests used in gastroenterology.

Chapter objectives

After reading this chapter you should be able to:

- Describe the main diagnostic procedures and equipment used in gastro-enterology.
- Understand the rationale behind diagnostic procedures.
- Identify the role of appropriate investigations for the range of gastrointestinal disorders.
- Relate diagnostic procedures to clinical nursing practice.

ENDOSCOPY

Gastrointestinal endoscopy involves the direct visual examination of the lumen of the gastrointestinal tract. It is a relatively safe and effective way of evaluating the appearance and integrity of the gastrointestinal mucosa for the purpose of diagnosis and provides access for therapeutic procedures. The techniques for endoscopic investigations of the upper and lower gastrointestinal tract include gastroscopy (oesophogastroduodenoscopy), ERCP (endoscopic retrograde cholangiopancreatography), EUS (endoscopic ultrasonography), colonoscopy and flexible and rigid sigmoidoscopy.

Nurse endoscopists

The British Society of Gastroenterology (BSG) Working Party (1994) gave support to the establishment of nurse endoscopists. Their report highlighted the potential role for nurses to perform gastrointestinal endoscopy as long as adequate training for all procedures is available (BSG 1994). The BSG proposed the role of the nurse endoscopist to complement and increase the capacity of existing medical endoscopy teams.

The NMC document *The Scope of Professional Practice* (NMC 2002) supports nurses in role development, for example carrying out gastrointestinal endoscopy. In addition, the nursing profession in the UK established the frameworks necessary to allow the development of nursing roles into areas once dominated by the medical profession (DoH 1997).

Because of the risks associated with therapeutic endoscopy the BSG working party considered that the nurse endoscopist's work should be confined to diagnostic gastroscopy with or without biopsy, and flexible sigmoidoscopy with or without biopsy. All therapeutic procedures, ERCP and colonoscopy are excluded from the endoscopist's remit. Understandable concern has been expressed by nurses with respect to the potential legal implications of endoscopic practice and the need for full medico-legal cover in the event of complications. Damage to teeth, bridges, crowns and other expensive dental treatments may be a potential source of litigation. The working party aimed to tackle these philosophical and practical issues and summarised:

- There is an increasing demand from within both the medical and nursing professions to perform endoscopy.
- Medico-legally, nurses may perform an endoscopy provided they have received appropriate training and are adequately supervised by a responsible consultant.
- Careful patient selection is essential to exclude high-risk patients and those requiring therapeutic procedures.
- A designated medical endoscopist should be immediately available during nurse endoscopy sessions.
- The nurse should be responsible for obtaining consent from the patient before endoscopy and for discussing the findings with the patient after the procedure (BSG 1999).
- The nurse should be responsible for preparing and signing the endoscopy report.
- Regular records and audit of the nurse endoscopist's work should take place.
- Continuing education is essential, with regular opportunities to attend endoscopy courses and meetings.

Under these described circumstances the BSG working party gave support to the proposal that nurses perform endoscopy.

Current best practice guidelines on sedation for endoscopy are published by the BSG (2003).

Endoscopy is clearly an area in which nurses are being encouraged to extend their practice into invasive and diagnostic techniques. Such procedures are anxiety-provoking for patients, who remain conscious throughout, and nurses are uniquely positioned to provide the technical expertise and the psychosocial support required. The extension of practice into endoscopy demonstrates two aspects of nursing which are increasingly coming to the fore: the extent to which nurses require detailed knowledge of anatomy, physiology and pathology and the issue of accountability.

In terms of the knowledge required, nothing less than a deep knowledge of the relevant areas of the gastrointestinal tract is required. Nurses cannot simply carry out such procedures by rote; they need to know what is normal and what is abnormal and if they are to provide the holistic care which is increasingly expected of them, they need to be sufficiently educated in the whole field of gastroenterology in order to explain procedures fully to patients and to discuss likely diagnoses and outcomes.

In terms of accountability, the issue of education is also raised: how can a nurse perform a procedure, with attendant risks and the potential for psychological morbidity, without being fully aware of the significance of each action they are performing? If nurses are to carry out advanced procedures under an extended role, they must be willing and able to be accountable for all aspects of the procedures they are undertaking. This chapter outlines the likely roles and responsibilities of nurse endoscopists and it is hoped that those who seek this role will extend their knowledge at the same time as extending their practice.

Types of endoscopes

Depending upon the area of the gastrointestinal tract that is required to be seen there are a range of endoscopes that can be used:

- A flexible end-viewing or side-viewing (oblique) endoscope – to view the oesophagus, stomach and proximal duodenum.
- A colonoscope, which is a 120–180 cm flexible endoscope – to view the entire lower gastrointestinal tract.
- A flexible sigmoidoscope, which may be up to 65 cm in length – to examine the rectum and the sigmoid and descending colon.
- An anoscope, which is a rigid plastic or metal speculum – for inspection of the anal canal.
- A proctosigmoidoscope, which is a 15–25 cm rigid endoscope – to examine the rectum and sigmoid colon.

Although all these instruments are designed for specific uses, all endoscopes have several common features, which include the following:

- A flexible insertion tube which is usually 8–12 mm in diameter. This insertion tube contains air, water and biopsy channels, and fibre bundles.
- An umbilical cord that extends from the control head and leads to the light source.
- An optic system, which consists of fibreoptic bundles that conduct light through the shaft and transmit the images to the eye. In video endoscope,

the optic system consists of a one-piece video camera that transmits images directly to a television screen with no need for fibreoptics.
- A control head that houses the lenses, controls for manoeuvring the tip up and down and from side to side, and valves that regulate irrigation, air or carbon dioxide insufflation and suction.
- Channels for air and water flow.
- A suction/biopsy channel that allows the passage of accessory instruments, such as biopsy forceps, cytology brushes, polypectomy snares, laser fibres or stents. The suction channel also allows for suctioning fluid that obstructs the endoscopist's vision.

Gastroscopy

Gastroscopy, or oesophogastroduodenoscopy, uses a flexible endoscope less than 10 mm in diameter, which is passed directly into the upper gastrointestinal tract. The entire oesophagus and stomach and proximal duodenum can be visualised. Larger diameter gastroscopes with larger suction channels are used for therapeutic procedures.

Gastroscopy allows the physician or nurse endoscopist to diagnose and document gastrointestinal disorders through the use of direct vision and video photography.

Diagnostic gastroscopy is generally indicated for evaluating:

- dysphagia or odynophagia
- dyspepsia
- gastro-oesophageal reflux symptoms unresponsive to medical therapy
- haematemisis/melaena
- oesophageal or gastric varices
- oesophagitis or gastritis
- gastric and peptic ulcers
- chronic abdominal pain
- suspected polyps and cancer
- removal of ingested foreign bodies
- acute injury following caustic ingestion
- management of achalasia

Gastroscopy is generally not indicated for evaluating:

- symptoms which are considered functional in origin
- metastatic adenocarcinoma

Prior to gastroscopy, patients require thorough medical and nursing assessment with special attention given to any history of drug reactions, bleeding disorders or associated cardiac, pulmonary, renal or hepatic disease.

Nursing care during gastroscopy

During gastroscopy the nursing responsibilities include the maintenance of the patient's oral airway, suctioning secretions and regurgitated material when necessary from the pharynx. Nasal oxygen should be used to treat hypoxia, and resuscitation equipment should be immediately available in the event of cardiopulmonary complications. The nurse should monitor the patient's oxygen saturation and vital signs regularly and observe the patient for signs of bleeding, vomiting, change in vital signs, pain and abdominal distension. Patients should be fasted for at least four hours prior to gastroscopy, longer if they have eaten a large meal.

Although gastroscopy is generally regarded as a safe procedure, adverse events can occur, including:

- respiratory depression
- effects of sedation
- perforation of the oesophagus, stomach or duodenum
- haemorrhage related to trauma and perforation
- pulmonary aspiration of blood or secretions, or regurgitation of gastric contents
- cardiac arrhythmia
- infection
- allergic reaction to the anaesthetic or intravenous medications

The rate of adverse events and complications increases when therapeutic manoeuvres are performed. Patients at the highest risk during gastroscopy are older people and those with advanced cardiac, pulmonary, hepatic or central nervous system disease.

Endoscopic retrograde cholangiopancreatography (ERCP)

ERCP uses a combination of endoscopic and radiological techniques to visualise the biliary and pancreatic ducts. It involves the injection of a contrast material into the biliary and pancreatic systems followed by radiological screening. Two different contrasts are used: low iodine for the common bile duct and higher iodine contrast for the pancreatic duct.

ERCP is indicated for the following:

- Signs and symptoms of pancreatic malignancy.
- Evaluation of acute, recurrent pancreatitis.
- Removal of retained common bile duct stones.
- Unexplained chronic abdominal pain of suspected biliary or pancreatic origin.

- Evaluation of patients with jaundice.
- Pre-operative or post-operative evaluation to detect common duct stones in patients who undergo laparoscopic cholecystectomy.

Prior to ERCP, patients should be fasted for six hours. Barium studies should not be conducted within 72 hours preceding ERCP because the residual barium can obstruct the view of the contrast medium in the ducts. As ERCP can be a longer procedure than gastroscopy, higher levels of sedation and analgesia are usually required.

The patient should be positioned in either the prone or left lateral position prior to the procedure. A side-viewing duodenoscope is passed by the endoscopist into the second part of the duodenum. Glucagon may be injected intravenously to suppress duodenal peristalsis and thereby aid visualisation. When the scope is in the correct location to view the ampulla of Vater, the patient is moved into the prone position. The endoscopist passes a plastic cannula through the endoscope and manoeuvres it into the orifice of the ampulla. Once the cannula is in the pancreatic duct or the common bile duct, the radiocontrast material is injected. The patient should be closely monitored for any reaction to the radiocontrast dye.

Nursing responsibilities during ERCP

The main responsibilities of the nurse during ERCP are:

- Assess, monitor, and document oxygen saturation and vital signs.
- Observe the patient for signs of abdominal distension.
- Maintain the patient's airway until the gag reflex returns.
- Observe for signs of pancreatitis, low-grade fever, pain, vomiting and tachycardia.
- Administer antibiotics as prescribed. ERCP may introduce infection leading to cholangitis, therefore prophylactic antibiotics are given to patients with biliary or pancreatic stasis.

Following the procedure, the patient's temperature should be checked every four hours for 48 hours. The most significant complications associated with ERCP are pancreatitis and sepsis.

Injury to the pancreas can result from chemical, enzymatic, mechanical, microbiological or hydrostatic factors. In patients with partial obstruction of either the pancreatic or common bile duct, a frequent complication of ERCP is biliary sepsis. The introduction of infection into a stagnant duct system can result in cholangitis and septicaemia. Additional potential complications include aspiration, bleeding, perforation, respiratory depression or arrest and cardiac arrythmias or arrest. Acute pancreatitis is caused in about 1% of ERCPs (Imrie 2000).

Proctosigmoidoscopy

Proctosigmoidoscopy is an examination of the rectum and sigmoid colon using a proctoscope, a rigid tube with a detachable, disposable end which is used for one patient only and then discarded. The proctoscope is 25–30 cm in length and approximately 1.5 cm in diameter. Proctosigmoidoscopy gives valuable information about the anal canal and rectum, but as the instrument is rigid it cannot be used to view above the splenic flexure. Indications for proctosigmoidoscopy include:

- melaena
- persistent diarrhoea
- passage of mucus and pus with stool
- bacteriology or histological studies
- rectal pain

Preparation involves a hypertonic phosphate enema on the morning of the procedure, to clean out the large bowel. Sedation is rarely required for proctosigmoidoscopy. The patient is asked to lie on his or her left side with knees drawn up to the chest, the scope is gently inserted, the obturator is removed, and air is pumped through the protosigmoidoscope to inflate the rectum. The examiner will note the colour and friability of the rectal mucosa, and bleeding sites and ulcers. Throughout the procedure the nurse should monitor the patient's vital signs, abdominal distension, pain tolerance and the condition of the skin.

Flexible sigmoidoscopy

Flexible sigmoidoscopy employs a flexible instrument to examine the rectum, sigmoid and a variable length of more proximal colon. The flexible sigmoidoscope measures up to 65 cm in length and its flexibility allows the endoscopist to reach the descending colon in up to 80% of patients. One additional benefit of flexible sigmoidoscopy is that it is better tolerated than rigid protosigmoidoscopy in many patients. Flexible sigmoidoscopy is generally indicated for:

- Screening of asymptomatic patients at risk of colonic cancer.
- Evaluation of suspected distal colonic disease when there is no indication for colonoscopy.
- Evaluation of the colon in conjunction with radiological examinations.
- Patients with a family history of colorectal cancer.
- Flexible sigmoidoscopy is generally not indicated when colonoscopy is indicated.

Contraindications for flexible sigmoidoscopy are similar to those listed for colonoscopy and should be avoided in documented acute diverticulitis.

Colonoscopy

Colonoscopy gives information about the lower gastrointestinal tract and is performed to examine the entire colon and rectum, almost always under sedation. Modern colonoscopes are similar in design to upper gastrointestinal endoscopes but are longer, ranging from 1.2 to 1.8 m.

Diagnostic colonoscopy is indicated in the following situations:

- Evaluation of active or occult lower gastrointestinal bleeding.
- Unexplained faecal occult blood.
- Unexplained iron deficiency anaemia.
- Confirmation of suspected polyps or strictures.
- Surveillance for colorectal cancer.
- Screening of patients with family history of colorectal cancer.
- Diagnosis and evaluation of chronic inflammatory bowel disease.
- Surveillance of long-term ulcerative colitis patients.
- Treatment of a bleeding lesion (e.g. laser or injection therapy).
- Palliative treatment of neoplasm (e.g. laser or stenting).
- Foreign body removal.

Colonoscopy is generally not indicated in the following circumstances:

- Acute diarrhoea.
- Routine follow-up of inflammatory bowel disease (except cancer surveillance in long-standing ulcerative colitis).
- Upper gastrointestinal bleed or melaena with a demonstrated upper gastrointestinal source.

Preparation of the bowel to enable a successful colonoscopy is vital. The presence of small particles of faecal matter may obscure the endoscopist's view of the colonic mucosa, therefore thorough bowel preparation is essential to avoid the patient having repeat colonoscopies. Bowel preparation is achieved by restricting diet to a low residue or clear fluid intake the day before the procedure. There are a range of purgatives available for patients to take in advance of their procedure; this usually involves administration of large volumes (several litres) of an isoomolar electrolyte lavage solution. The patient may benefit from being informed that the preparation can be the most unpleasant part of the procedure, but that it is vital for a successful examination.

The nurse will have several responsibilities in the patient preparation for colonoscopy, including:

- Recording of baseline vital signs so that abnormalities can be detected during the procedure.
- Obtaining informed consent.
- Giving the patient the opportunity to urinate prior to the procedure.
- Fasting the patient for several hours before the procedure to prevent the risk of aspiration during sedation.

The nurse caring for the patient following a colonoscopy should be aware that the patient will still be drowsy after the procedure and should be allowed to sleep until their sedation wears off before being offered a drink. Vital signs (pulse, blood pressure and rate of respiration) must be recorded regularly (every 15 minutes) following the procedure to allow detection of signs of any abnormalities, noting risk of perforation to the bowel or oversedation. Major complications occur in less than 1% of patients undergoing colonoscopy. The two main complications, perforation and haemorrhage, usually occur after the removal of polyps – polypectomy. It is important that the nurse is aware of any signs of complications, such as bleeding, vomiting, abdominal pain and rigidity, and that these are recorded.

Small bowel enteroscopy

Enteroscopy allows the visualisation of a greater extent of the small bowel than gastroscopy. There are two types of enteroscopes available: the push enteroscope, which allows limited tissue sampling and therapy, and the sonde enteroscope, which potentially allows the entire small bowel to be seen without the possibility of therapeutic intervention.

Enteroscopy is generally indicated for:

- Evaluation of the source of gastrointestinal bleeding not identified by gastroscopy or colonoscopy.
- Evaluation of an abnormal radiological image of the small bowel.
- Localisation of known or suspected small bowel lesions.
- Therapy (with push enteroscope) of small bowel lesions.

If the source of bleeding can be identified with gastroscopy or colonoscopy, enteroscopy is generally not indicated.

Endoscopic ultrasound

Advances in technology have led to the combination of endoscopes with ultrasonography to enhance visualisation of the gastrointestinal tract. This technique is called endoscopic ultrasound (EUS) and allows for better quality resolution, which enhances evaluation of structures. The walls of the oesophagus, stomach, duodenum and colon can be visualised, as well as the structure of several adjacent organs.

The general indications for EUS include:

- Staging tumours of the gastrointestinal tract, pancreas and bile ducts.
- Evaluating abnormalities of the gastrointestinal tract wall or adjacent structures.
- Sampling of tissue lesions within, or adjacent to, the wall of the gastrointestinal tract.
- Evaluation of abnormalities of the pancreas and biliary tree.
- Providing endoscopic therapy under ultrasonographic guidance.

Although developing, the role of EUS, as compared with endoscopic and radiological examinations, has a greater ability to detect lesions in the wall of the gastrointestinal tract.

DIAGNOSTIC TESTS AND PROCEDURES IN GASTROENTEROLOGY

The remainder of this chapter examines a number of tests and procedures that nurses will encounter in gastrointestinal medicine. These tests and procedures are available to confirm or disprove diagnoses. Endoscopic procedures have been covered earlier in this chapter. Radiological studies and tests involving the analysis of blood, urine and faeces are reviewed in this section.

It is vital for the nurse to understand the role of tests and investigations that are undertaken in gastroenterology as the nurse will be involved in the preparation and education of patients. Research has shown that patient anxiety can be reduced and patient compliance improved if nurses provide appropriate information and education prior to a procedure.

Radiological investigations

Radiological studies such as barium swallow, barium enema and gastrointestinal upper series are used in gastroenterology to detect abnormalities of the gastrointestinal tract. Barium studies are in general more easily tolerated than endoscopic investigations and have fewer complications; however, endoscopy has a greater diagnostic potential.

Most radiological studies use barium as a contrast medium. This is a chalky, non-allergenic substance that allows for X-ray examination of the oesophagus, stomach and lower gastrointestinal tract. The barium preparation is usually administered orally or rectally and its use is contraindicated in patients with suspected gastrointestinal obstruction or perforation. The nurse should caution the patient to report failure to pass the barium within 48 hours so that appropriate measures, an enema or laxative, can be initiated to avoid constipation or obstruction.

Barium swallow

Barium swallow allows for radiological examination of the oesophagus. This procedure can reveal the presence or absence of strictures, motility disorders, ulceration and foreign bodies. As a diagnostic tool, barium swallow is less sensitive than endoscopy; if possible, barium swallow should be avoided in patients with dysphagia.

Upper gastrointestinal series

Radiological examination of the stomach and small intestine involves ingestion of a barium solution followed by an upper gastrointestinal series with small bowel follow-through. This procedure allows for diagnosis of diverticula, strictures, hiatus hernia, motility disorders and tumours. Upper gastrointestinal series is also used in the examination of Crohn's disease and malabsorption syndromes.

Barium enema

Barium enema allows radiological examination of the colon. It is a common test used for the detection of polyps, diverticula and structural changes in the colon, and may be used for the diagnosis of colorectal cancer and inflammatory bowel diseases.

Abdominal ultrasound

Abdominal ultrasound is a non-invasive procedure that can indicate the size and shape of organs. It can detect any abnormalities of structures or spaces within the abdominal cavity through the transmission of sound waves. Abdominal ultrasound may be useful for initial detection of gallstones, as it involves minimal patient preparation and no radiation. Ultrasound investigations can also be used to diagnose acute cholecystitis.

Computed tomography (CT) scan

CT scanners have been used since the 1970s and produce computerised images of the body in a series of cross-sectional views. CT scanning is a non-invasive, radiological scanning technique that involves the measurement of differences in tissue density to reflect tissue configuration. CT scanning

Table 10.1 Approximate reference ranges.

Red blood cell (RBC)	Males $4.5-6.5 \times 10^{12}/l$
	Females $3.9-5.6 \times 10^{12}/l$
Haemoglobin (Hb)	Males $13.5-17.5$ g/dl
	Females $11.5-15.5$ g/dl
Haematocrit (Ht)	Males $40-52\%$
	Females $36-48\%$
Mean cell haemoglobin concentration (MCHC) $20-35$ g/dl	
Critical values	
Haemoglobin	< 7.0 g/dl or > 20.0 g/dl

produces a three-dimensional image which is more detailed and accurate than images produced by abdominal ultrasound. CT scans are commonly used for detection of malignancy in the gall bladder and pancreas.

Blood tests in gastrointestinal medicine

This is a brief overview of the more commonly used blood tests. Reference ranges are provided in Table 10.1.

Haemoglobin/haematocrit

Haemoglobin is the oxygen-carrying pigment of red cells, and haematocrit refers to the volume percentage of erythrocytes in whole blood. Levels of both haemoglobin and haematocrit are influenced by pathology in the gastrointestinal tract and will decrease when a patient is anaemic, such as during a gastrointestinal bleed.

Platelet count

Platelet count is a count of the number of platelets present in blood. A low platelet count would be indicative of impaired clotting mechanisms.

Prothrombin level/time

Prothrombin is a glycoprotein present in blood plasma that is normally converted to thrombin. Impaired absorption of vitamin K from the intestine can result in decreased prothrombin levels. Low prothrombin levels are seen in a patient's liver and in small bowel disease. Prothrombin time relates to the measurement of blood clotting. Prolonged prothrombin times are seen in patients who are unable to absorb vitamin K, and in individuals with poor nutrition, liver disease and blood disorders.

Liver function tests

Liver function tests may be carried out on blood, urine and faeces to detect the levels of substances manufactured by the liver as well as to estimate other functions of the liver (i.e. excretion). Liver function tests are usually defined as the measurement of serum levels of:

- albumin
- bilirubin
- aminotransferase
- alkaline phosphotase
- γ-glutamyltransferase

Serum albumin

Serum albumin is a good indicator of chronic liver disease. It is synthesised by the liver and its levels fall in chronic liver disease.

Conclusion

Nurses working in gastroenterology are increasingly being enabled, through specialist and nationally recognised courses, to undertake training and extend their practice as nurse endoscopists. These developments are in line with UK government policy, which seeks to extend the clinical capabilities of nurses generally and also in line with the development of the nurse consultant role.

Extending nursing practice into invasive and diagnostic procedures such as endoscopy raises several issues for nurses, including accountability, relationships with the medical and surgical professions and the knowledge base required for such practice. It is already clear that nurses are able to carry out endoscopy safely and it is likely that there will be a major expansion in this role. In addition to being able to undertake this devolved medical procedure, nurses are ideally placed to undertake it as these invasive procedures are associated with a great deal of anxiety in patients regarding the procedure itself and the possible outcome in terms of diagnosis – especially of malignant conditions. The nurse endoscopist, in addition to performing the endoscopy, is able to offer support through detailed and clear explanations to the patient of what they are likely to experience, and for minor conditions such as haemorrhoids can carry out certain treatments and offer ongoing advice about diet and lifestyle which may help to alleviate further problems. Nurses should also have a thorough understanding of the medical and surgical roles in relation to the possible outcomes of endoscopy or the need for further, more invasive procedures which they are not competent to carry out.

However, the most important aspect of the preparation of nurse endoscopists is the knowledge of the relevant anatomy and physiology of the gastrointestinal tract that is required. This must be beyond the superficial aspects of structure, function and control and must incorporate the pathology and pathophysiology of gastrointestinal disorder to ensure that nurses can offer the right kind of support to patients and liaison with medical and surgical colleagues, and can be truly accountable for every aspect of their extended role.

BACKGROUND READING

Additional reading to support the material in this chapter can be found in the relevant sections of the following texts:

Alexander, M., Fawcett, J.N. and Runciman, P. (2000) *Nursing Practice: Hospital and Home – the Adult*. Churchill Livingstone, Edinburgh (Chapter 4).

Brooker, C. and Nicol, M. (2003) *Nursing Adults: the Practice of Caring*. Mosby, London (Chapter 22).

Clancy, J., McVicar, A.J. and Baird, N. (2002) *Perioperative Practice: Fundamentals of Homeostasis*. Routledge, London (Chapter 2).

Haslett, C., Chilvers, E.R., Boon, N.A. and Colledge, N.R. (2002) *Davidson's Principles and Practice of Medicine*, 19th edition. Churchill Livingstone, Edinburgh (Chapter 17).

Higgins, C. (2000) *Understanding Laboratory Investigations: a Text for Nurses and Healthcare Professionals*. Blackwell Publishing, Oxford.

Walsh, M. (2002) *Clinical Nursing and Related Sciences*, 6th edition. Ballière Tindall, London (Chapter 9).

BEST PRACTICE GUIDELINES

BSG (2003) *Safety and Sedation During Endoscopic Procedures* (http://www.bsg.org.uk/clinical_prac/guidelines/sedation.htm accessed 8 May 2004).

REFERENCES

British Society of Gastroenterology Working Party (1994) *The Nurse Endoscopist*. British Society of Gastroenterology, Glasgow (http://www.bsg.org.uk/clinical_prac/guidelines/nurse_endo.htm accessed 8 May 2004).

BSG (1999) *Guidelines for Informed Consent for Endoscopic Procedures* (http://www.bsg.org.uk/clinical_prac/guidelines/consent.htm accessed 8 May 2004).

DoH (1997) *The Extending Role of the Clinical Nurse*. Legal Implications and Training Requirements, Vol. 22 (HO 77). Department of Health, London.

Imrie, C.W. (2000) Acute pancreatitis. In: *Concise Oxford Textbook of Medicine* (Leadingham, J.G.G. and Worrell, D.A., eds), pp. 600–603. Oxford University Press, Oxford.

NMC (2002) *The Scope of Professional Practice*. Nursing and Midwifery Council, London.

Chapter 11
Gastrointestinal Emergencies

Chapter objectives

After reading this chapter you should be able to:

- Describe the underlying pathophysiology of common gastrointestinal emergencies.
- Understand the cause and risk factors of gastrointestinal emergencies.
- Identify the main symptoms of complications.
- Relate the measures that are required to treat gastrointestinal emergencies, and the relevant nursing practice.

Perforation of the gastrointestinal tract

Perforation of the gastrointestinal tract can occur in the oesophagus, stomach or duodenum. It can be the result of trauma, underlying pathology, ingestion of a foreign body, increased intraoesophageal pressure or mechanical trauma during upper endoscopy. Oesophageal perforation during therapeutic upper endoscopy most commonly occurs during dilatation of oesophageal strictures. It can also be the result of instrument trauma during an endoscopic procedure, caused by the instrument, dilators or biopsy forceps. Gastric perforation is less common than oesophageal perforation and is usually related to peptic ulcer disease.

Clinical presentation of gastrointestinal perforation

The most common presenting symptom is pain. This pain and other presenting signs and symptoms are dictated by the site and severity of the perforation.

Oesophageal perforation

If the perforation is in the upper third of the oesophagus the patient will have dysphagia, stiffness of the neck and tenderness in the region affected. Perforation in the thoracic oesophagus can result in sub-sternal or epigastric pain that is increased with respirations and movement. In the distal region of the oeso-phagus a perforation may result in shoulder pain, dyspnea, severe back and abdominal pain, tachycardia, cyanosis and hypotension.

Sudden chest pain after vomiting is the cardinal symptom when the distal posterior oesophageal wall tears longitudinally in a spontaneous perforation, called Boorhaeve's syndrome.

Duodenal perforation

After a duodenal perforation the vital signs may remain stable for a time. This is usually followed by the experience of sudden, local, abdominal pain. Duo-denal perforation can lead to the development of peritonitis. The patient's abdomen becomes rigid and fever develops.

Perforation of the lower gastrointestinal tract

Lower gastrointestinal perforations can be either spontaneous or mechanical. Conditions such as inflammatory bowel disease, ischaemic colitis, adhesions, strictures, diverticular disease or malignancy are believed to put patients at higher risk. Lower gastrointestinal perforations occur most often from mechanical trauma related to the manipulation of the endoscopic instrument during colonoscopy.

Pneumatic perforation may result from overdistension with insufflated air. The risk of perforation is almost doubled in polypectomy with dia-gnostic colonoscopy and is usually related to electrical injury of the bowel wall. Several predisposing factors can increase the risk of post-polypectomy perforation, often related to large polyps. Signs of a lower gastrointestinal perforation include sudden, severe, abdominal pain accompanied by signs of peritonitis, abdominal distension, malaise, a change in vital signs and fever. Perforation of the colon may be seen by the endoscopist or diagnosed by a radiographer using plain abdominal radiography with the patient in the supine position.

Gastrointestinal haemorrhage

Frank gastrointestinal bleeding is very distressing for patients, especially from the upper tract, and the nurse has an important role to play in remaining calm and reassuring the patient about any action that needs to be taken. This, combined with good first-aid skills, will save lives and lead to effective treat-ment of any underlying gastrointestinal conditions.

In general, bright red blood comes from low in the tract, and dark, altered blood from higher up the gastrointestinal tract. However, profuse bleeding from the upper gut may produce too much blood to be altered on its way through the tract and it may appear red.

Box 11.1   Some common causes of upper gastrointestinal bleed in adults.

- Duodenal and gastric ulceration
- Oesophagitis
- Gastritis
- Duodenitis
- Oesophageal varices
- Mallory-Weiss tear
- Carcinoma

Gastrointestinal haemorrhage may be associated with an underlying clinical condition or trauma or may result as a rare complication of diagnostic endoscopy.

Complications of gastrointestinal haemorrhage include:

- anaemia from blood loss
- exsanguination from rapid massive intravascular blood loss
- hypovolaemic shock from severe volume depletion
- aspiration in upper gastrointestinal bleed
- myocardial or cerebral infarction from acute haemoglobin depletion
- disseminated intravascular coagulation from shock and clotting factor loss
- peritonitis and sepsis from bowel rupture

Upper gastrointestinal haemorrhage

Acute upper gastrointestinal bleed is one of the most common medical emergencies. The most common causes of upper gastrointestinal bleeding are listed in Box 11.1. Peptic ulceration accounts for up to a half of all cases of upper gastrointestinal bleeding. These ulcers are defects in the gastrointestinal mucosa which relate to the activity of pepsin and gastric acid. The three most common categories of ulcers are ulcers related to *Helicobacter pylori* infection, ulcers caused by NSAIDs (i.e. aspirin) and stress ulcers.

Upper gastrointestinal bleeding is usually indicated by haematemesis, hypotension, tachycardia and melaena.

Precipitating factors for upper gastrointestinal bleeds include:

- traumatisation of recently bleeding oesophageal varices
- oesophagitis
- gastritis
- duodenitis
- mucosal tear in patients with strictures
- Mallory-Weiss (cardio-oesophageal) tear
- peptic ulcer disease

In an acute upper gastrointestinal bleed, upper endoscopy may reveal stigmata of recent haemorrhage, such as a visible vessel, fresh blood clot or active bleeding. If no signs of recent haemorrhage are visible, medical therapy may be sufficient. In patients with continued bleeding or stigmata of recent haemorrhage, therapeutic endoscopy may be indicated.

Resuscitation of upper gastrointestinal bleeding
The main initial priority in management of a patient with a gastrointestinal bleed is to resuscitate the patient and preserve oxygenation of vital organs. The patient will be assessed for clues to the cause of the haemorrhage and for signs of shock; these are discussed below.

Best practice guidelines for the management of non-variceal haemorrhage have been published by BSG (2002).

Lower gastrointestinal bleeding

Common causes of lower gastrointestinal bleeding are:

- diverticulosis
- inflammatory bowel disease
- colonic angiodysplasia
- haemorrhoids

Massive bleeding from the lower gastrointestinal tract is relatively uncommon. The most common causes of lower gastrointestinal bleeding are minor anorectal conditions, such as haemorroids. Other common causes of lower gastrointestinal bleeding include colorectal polyps, colorectal carcinoma and ulcerative colitis. Drug therapy can also cause rectal bleeding (usually occult); in particular, non-steroidal anti-inflammatory drugs (NSAIDs) can lead to small bowel enteropathy and anti-coagulant therapy may provoke bleeding from minor mucosal lesions or malignancies. Lower gastrointestinal bleed is associated with symptoms of increased pulse rate, decreased blood pressure, weakness and black stools.

Colonoscopy is essential to determine the site of bleeding in a lower gastrointestinal bleed. This will allow exclusion of angiodysplasia and will prevent inappropriate surgery being performed.

Nurses involved in the assessment of a patient with a suspected gastrointestinal haemorrhage may undertake the following:

- History of presenting symptoms, including haemetemesis, pain and abdominal tenderness.
- History of concomitant heart, lung, renal, liver or central nervous system (CNS) disease.
- Recording of vital signs.
- Physical examination (including rectal examination).

Investigations for lower gastrointestinal bleed include:

- Rectal examination: digital examination to palpate rectal lesions.
- Proctoscopy: the distal rectum can be examined for haemorrhoids.
- Sigmoidoscopy: flexible or rigid sigmoidoscopy can examine the sigmoid colon.
- Barium enema: to detect mucosal lesions.
- Angiography: to demonstrate vascular abnormalities, e.g. angiodysplasia.
- Colonoscopy: allows for early diagnosis and treatment of polyps.

Management of a gastrointestinal bleed

The initial management of the patient with an upper gastrointestinal bleed should focus on maintaining the airway, providing oxygenation, establishing intravenous access, maintaining adequate fluid volume, stabilising the patient's condition, stopping the source of bleeding and commencing appropriate therapy to prevent rebleeding. Prompt endoscopic examination may be indicated to make a diagnosis and stop bleeding.

Shock

Shock is defined as a condition of acute peripheral circulatory failure caused by derangement of circulatory control or loss of circulatory fluid. It is characterised by decreased tissue perfusion and increased peripheral vasoconstriction. In gastroenterology, the two most common forms of shock are hypovolaemic shock and bacterial (septic) shock.

Hypovolaemic shock

In hypovolaemic shock, the loss of circulating volume may be the consequence of loss of blood or plasma, intestinal obstruction, nephrotic syndrome, dehydration or trauma. Hypovolaemia causes the body to adapt to the volume loss by decreasing urinary output and vasoconstriction of peripheral blood vessels. Glycogen breakdown increases, insulin is suppressed and hyperglycaemia can occur.

Common signs and symptoms of hypovolaemic shock are:

- tachycardia
- restlessness
- increased anxiety
- pale, cool, clammy skin
- decreased capillary refill time (noted by pressing on the fingernail)

In the early stages of hypovolaemic shock hypertension may occur. Hypotension is an advanced sign. The main principles of treatment in the hypovolaemic patient focus on restoring tissue perfusion and reducing peripheral vasoconstriction. The nurse should ensure that the patient is positioned in a way that promotes blood supply to the brain and venous return to the rest of the body.

Intravenous fluids should be administered to maintain the patency of the vascular system, to restore volume and an oxygen transport system and to remove wastes. The fluid given may be blood, plasma, plasma expander or a balanced salt solution, the choice of fluid depending on the patient's haematocrit levels.

Steroids may be given to decrease peripheral resistance, increase tissue perfusion, increase venous return and have a positive effect on heart muscle. Metabolic acidosis (the depletion of the body's alkali reserve, with resulting disturbance to the acid-base balance) is generally corrected with the administration of appropriate fluids.

Septic shock

Septic shock is produced by direct invasion of the bloodstream by micro-organisms or their toxins. Septic shock is usually associated with peritonitis, infections, bowel surgery, trauma or haemorrhage.

Initial signs of septic shock are:

- rigor/chills
- fever
- warm, flushed skin
- hypotension
- increased cardiac output

Without treatment, septic shock can rapidly progress towards the symptoms exhibited in hypovolaemic shock. Management involves removal of the cause, antibiotic therapy and prevention of system failure.

Conclusion

Emergencies arising from the gastrointestinal tract invariably involve bleeding and the possible consequence of shock. It is also clear that such emergencies commonly occur during routine gastrointestinal investigations involving endoscopy. The increasing development of nurse endoscopists means that nurses may increasingly, albeit inadvertently, be the cause of a gastrointestinal bleed and they need to be able to recognise the signs and take first-aid action.

BACKGROUND READING

Additional reading to support the material in this chapter can be found in the relevant sections of the following texts:

Haslett, C., Chilvers, E.R., Boon, N.A. and Colledge, N.R. (2002) *Davidson's Principles and Practice of Medicine*, 19th edition. Churchill Livingstone, Edinburgh (Chapter 17).

Kumar, P. and Clark, M. (2002) *Clinical Medicine*, 4th edition. Saunders, Edinburgh (Chapters 6 and 7).

BEST PRACTICE GUIDELINES

BSG (2002) Guidelines for Non-variceal Upper Gastrointestinal Haemorrhage (http://www.bsg.org.uk/clinical_prac/guidelines/nonvariceal.htm accessed 8 May 2004).

Chapter 12
Pharmacology in Gastroenterology

Chapter objectives

After reading this chapter you should be able to:

- Understand the principal types of drugs used in gastroenterology, especially:
    - The use of histamine H_2-receptor antagonists and proton pump inhibitors in the treatment of ulcer disease.
    - The use of antacid preparations in the treatment of GORD and dyspepsia.
    - The use of digestive enzymes in medical therapy.
    - Pharmaceutical management of constipation and diarrhoea.
    - Pharmaceutical management of inflammatory bowel disease and irritable bowel syndrome.

Drugs are prescribed to gastroenterology patients for a variety of reasons, to alter gastrointestinal secretion and motility. Pharmaceutical agents in gastroenterology may be administered orally, parenterally or topically. The route of administration is usually determined by the required speed of onset of the drug's effect, patient comfort and safety considerations, and the organ targeted by the drug. When the gastrointestinal system is the target of drug therapy, oral administration is often the most effective.

Administration of drugs

Oral medication

Oral medications can take the form of tablets, capsules, syrups, elixirs, liquids, suspensions, powders or granules. Most oral medications are swallowed by mouth, but they may also be given via a nasogastric or gastrostomy tube. Oral administration of medication can be contraindicated by nausea, vomiting, dysphagia or unconsciousness.

Parenteral route

This indicates administration of medication by injection, using a subcutaneous, intramuscular or intravenous route. The subcutaneous route provides a faster route than oral administration. Intramuscular injections deposit medication deep into the muscle tissue, where it can be readily absorbed.

Topical route

Depending upon their purpose, topical drugs may be administered to gastroenterology patients in the form of rectal suppositories, rectally administered foams and enemas, transdermal patches and ointments or sprays.

Types of drugs

Drugs used on the gastrointestinal tract vary widely in nature and pharmacological properties. They will be considered here under the headings of antacids, antibiotics, ulcer-healing agents, anti-emetics, antidiarrheals and laxatives.

Antacids

Antacids are used to reduce gastric acidity and afford relief in gastritis, gastro-oesphageal reflux, dyspepsia and any form of hyperacidity. Antacids usually contain combinations of aluminium, calcium and magnesium salts. Unlike other anti-ulcer agents, they have no direct effect on gastric acid secretion and they do not coat or protect the mucous lining. They work by reducing the total acid load in the gastrointestinal tract by buffering the acid that is being produced, thereby raising the gastric pH. Antacids also strengthen the gastric mucosal barrier.

Although antacids can be used for peptic ulcer disease they have been superseded by proton-pump inhibitors and histamine H_2-receptor blocking agents.

Commonly used antacids in gastroenterology include:

- aluminium hydroxide
- calcium carbonate
- magnesium carbonate
- magnesium trisilicate
- sodium bicarbonate

Prolonged use of antacids containing magnesium or calcium may cause systemic absorption of toxic quantities of magnesium or calcium ions. Excessive use of aluminium-containing antacids may lead to hypophosphataemia. Antacids containing sodium can precipitate oedema in patients with liver disease, hypertension or congestive heart failure.

Antibiotics

Antibiotics are prescribed in gastroenterology for severe cases of infectious diarrhoea, Crohn's disease and treatment for bacterial infections, including *Helicobacter pylori*. Bacterial infectious organisms that respond to antibiotics include *Escherichia coli*, *Shigella*, *Helicobacter*, *Vibrio cholerae* and *Clostridium difficile*.

Antibiotics that are prescribed for patients with infectious diarrhoea are ampicillin, metranidazole, tetracycline and vancomycin. The specific drug prescribed depends upon the bacterial agent involved.

Ulcer-healing drugs

Peptic ulcers can result from autodigestion, which occurs when the natural defences, such as the protective mucous lining of the stomach and duodenum, are breached.

The various drugs prescribed for peptic ulcer disease promote healing by reducing gastric acid secretion, buffering secreted gastric acid and/or enhancing intrinsic mucosal defences. The classes of drugs used for these purposes include antacids, H_2 blockers, proton-pump inhibitors, anticholinergic agents and prostaglandins. Antacids have been discussed earlier in this chapter.

H_2 blockers include cimetidine and ranitidine. They reduce the secretion of gastric acid by blocking histamine's action on the H_2 receptors in the parietal cells. H_2 blockers may also reduce gastric acidity in patients with upper gastrointestinal bleeding that stems from a peptic ulcer.

Proton-pump inhibitors

Prostaglandins (i.e. misoprostal) have an antisecretory effect. They may be used to prevent gastric ulcers and mucosal injury that are associated with the use of non-steroidal anti-inflammatory drugs (NSAIDs). They have revolutionised the approach to management of gastrointestinal problems associated with hyperacidity. Their name relates to the process by which hydrochloric acid is formed in the parietal cells of the stomach (see Figure 12.1), which depends upon a supply of hydrogen ions (protons) being produced. There are now several proton-pump inhibitors available including omeprazole and lansoprazole.

Pancreatic enzymes

There are several gastrointestinal conditions that may result in a deficiency of pancreatic enzymes, including pancreatitis, cystic fibrosis and pancreatic duct obstruction. These conditions can lead to impairment of digestion resulting in

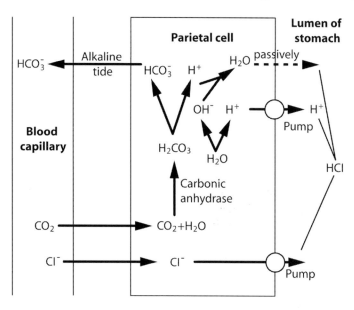

Figure 12.1 Formation of hydrochloric acid in the parietal cells of the stomach. Reproduced with permission from Hinchliff *et al.* (1996).

deficiencies of essential fatty acids. Patients with these disorders require supplemental pancreatic enzymes to ensure better digestion. Pancreatin is a preparation that includes a mixture of enzymes, including lipases, proteases and amylase. The main problem in prescribing pancreatic enzymes relates to their susceptibility to gastric acid. This can be overcome by giving the tablets an enteric coat.

Anti-emetics

Anti-emetics are drugs that prevent or modify nausea and vomiting. Anti-emetics comprise a diverse range of drugs, including dopamine receptor antagonists, antihistamines, anticholinergics, and 5HT$_3$ receptor antagonists.

Dopamine receptor antagonists are used to control nausea and vomiting. They antagonise dopamine receptors involved in the vomiting reflex, and they affect dopamine receptors in peripheral pathways, thereby increasing peristalsis and decreasing reflux, by facilitating gastric emptying. Dopamine receptor antagonists include metaclopramide, haloperidol, domperidone and prochlorperazine.

Antihistamines, including cyclizine, are a group of drugs that act directly on the H$_1$ receptors of the vomiting centre by antagonising the action of histamine. Antihistamines are the anti-emetic of choice when bowel obstruction, haemorrhage or perforation is suspected, so as to avoid the use of dopamine antagonists which increase bowel motility and therefore risk complications. The sedative side-effect is the main drawback related to the use of antihistamines.

Anticholinergics are commonly given as premedication, in order to dry bronchial and salivary secretions. These drugs have an antimuscarinic activity, with a depressant action on the vomiting centre and an antispasmodic action on the gastrointestinal tract. Hyoscine and atropine are examples of anticholinergics. Side-effects include dilation of the pupils, dry mouth and drowsiness. Anticholinergics may also be used in the treatment of peptic ulcer disease, irritable bowel syndrome, pancreatitis, gastritis and diffuse oesophageal spasm. Anticholinergic medications are contraindicated in older patients, who may be more susceptible to the central anticholinergic side-effects of dizziness, glaucoma and urinary retention.

The neurotransmitter serotonin, or $5HT_3$, is found in its highest concentration in the enterochromaffin cells of the intestinal mucosa. It has a variety of actions depending on the conditions and on its concentration. $5HT_3$ plays a role in the perceptions of pain, sleep and anxiety and in the nausea and vomiting reflex.

$5HT_3$ receptors are thought to activate the vagal nerve, and possibly the vomiting centre. They are easily administered either by mouth or intravenously, with minimal side-effects (headache and constipation).

Anti-emetic drugs should only be prescribed when the cause of vomiting is known, otherwise they may delay diagnosis.

Antidiarrhoeals

Antidiarrhoeal agents are used for symptomatic relief of diarrhoea. They include drugs that decrease intestinal motility and drugs that decrease the fluid content of the stool or inhibit intestinal secretions. Antidiarrhoeal agents can be used judiciously to treat symptoms in Crohn's disease, ulcerative colitis and irritable bowel syndrome.

Laxatives

Laxatives are used to induce defaecation. They are classified by their mechanisms of action. These include hyperosmotic colonic lavage solutions, which act by increasing intraluminal pressure to stimulate peristalsis. These solutions are composed of poorly absorbed solutes that cause the volume of chyme to increase by transport of water down the osmotic gradient into the lumen.

Stimulant cathartics act by producing local irritation and increasing intestinal motility. Bulk-forming cathartics are composed of natural or synthetic polysaccharides or cellulose derivatives that expand in the gut without being absorbed and therefore facilitate normal elimination. They consist of non-digestible cellulose fibres that become hydrated in the gut. This decreases the viscosity of the luminal contents to increase their flow through the intestines. Bulk-forming agents are generally the preferred treatment for constipation, as they are free from side-effects, relatively inexpensive and probably the most acceptable and natural of the treatment options for constipation. The addition of natural fibre and fruits to the diet provides a similar effect.

Emollient laxatives act as surfactants that soften the faecal mass by facilitating the mixture of aqueous and fatty substances. They increase the secretion of water in the small bowel and the colon. Examples of emollients are didactyl sodium sulphosuccinate and liquid paraffin. Liquid paraffin can interfere with the absorption of fat-soluble vitamins and so is rarely used.

Laxatives enemas are useful for softening impacted faeces and facilitating evacuation.

Laxatives may also be used to cleanse the bowel before colonoscopy, flexible sigmoidoscopy, barium studies or surgery. This enables elimination of substances from the gastrointestinal tract to facilitate the procedure.

Agents used in diagnostic tests

A number of different pharmacological agents may be used in the diagnosis of gastrointestinal disorders. Pentagastrin (peptavlon) is used to stimulate gastric acid secretion. Secretin is used in tests of pancreatic exocrine secretion. Glucagon is used in diagnostic and therapeutic procedures, primarily to reduce gastrointestinal motility.

Conclusion

Drugs play an important role in the management of gastrointestinal disorders. In fact, over-the-counter medications for mild gastrointestinal disorders are among the most commonly consumed drugs in the UK. Drugs have featured throughout this book and the purpose of this chapter is to provide some order to the subject in terms of the groups of drugs that are predominantly used to treat certain conditions.

A general awareness of the drugs used in gastroenterology is an essential adjunct to nursing practice in this area. However, with the advent of nurse prescribing and with some gastrointestinal system preparations included in the *Nurse Prescriber's Formulary*, it is essential that nurses are up to date in their knowledge of these drugs. Even for drugs which nurses are unlikely to prescribe, their knowledge should be up to date as they are often in the position of advising patients on their medication and explaining, for instance, why one preparation may have been prescribed over another.

Clearly, there are textbooks and formularies to which nurses, and doctors, can turn, but increasingly drug information is available on the World Wide Web and it is quite common for patients to access this information too. Nurses who are at the forefront of gastrointestinal practice, including nurse practitioners and nurse endoscopists, should be able to use the World Wide Web both to search for new information – and not just on drugs – and to update their knowledge of the drugs which are being used in practice. Two excellent websites at which information may be obtained are those of the National Institute for Clinical Excellence (NICE) (www.nice.org.uk/) and the British National Formulary (www.bnf.org.uk/bnf/).

BACKGROUND READING

Additional reading to support the material in this chapter can be found in the relevant sections of the following texts:

Haslett, C., Chilvers, E.R., Boon, N.A. and Colledge, N.R. (2002) *Davidson's Principles and Practice of Medicine*, 19th edition. Churchill Livingstone, Edinburgh (Chapters 17 and 18).

Kumar, P. and Clark, M. (2002) *Clinical Medicine*, 4th edition. Saunders, Edinburgh (Chapter 6 and 7).

McKenry, L.M. and Salerno, E. (1998) *Pharmacology for Nursing*, 20th edition. Mosby, St Louis.

Walsh, M. (2002) *Clinical Nursing and Related Sciences*, 6th edition. Baillière Tindall, London (Chapter 6).

Watson, R. (1999) *Essential Science for Nursing Students: an Introductory Text*. Baillière Tindall, London (Chapter 15).

Section 3
Living with Gastrointestinal Disorders

Chapter 13
The Role of Psychosocial Factors in Gastroenterology

Chapter objectives

After reading this chapter you should be able to:

- Be aware of psychosocial elements of gastroenterology.
- Understand:
    - The role of psychosocial factors in gastrointestinal illness.
    - Psychological intervention in gastroenterology.
    - The role of the nurse in psychosocial care.

Psychosocial factors play an important part in most gastrointestinal illnesses. Life stress, psychological state, coping and social support can be influential in the initial precipitation of illness and later exacerbations. Life stress refers to stressful life events, such as loss of job, breakup of a relationship, bereavement, sexual abuse or financial difficulties. Psychological state refers to the presence of psychiatric symptoms, such as depression or anxiety.

Anxiety and depression

Anxiety and depression are closely related and a combined state of both is common.

Anxiety

Anxiety is defined as a 'characteristic, unpleasant emotion induced by the anticipation of danger or frustration which threatens the security or homeostasis of the individual or the group to which he or she belongs'. Anxiety is associated with autonomic activation (fight or flight reaction), breathlessness, palpitations, chest or abdominal discomfort and diarrhoea.

Depression

Depression covers a wide range of psychological disturbances. There is little confusion about the recognition of a severe state of depression, but milder degrees of the condition can be difficult to recognise. Depressive states have been defined in terms of depressed mood, loss of interest, hopelessness, slowness and underactivity, inefficient thinking, poor concentration, suicidal plans or acts, morning depression, social withdrawal, guilt and observed depression. There are both emotional and physical aspects of these depressive states; the prime psychological symptom is lowering of mood with a persistent and prevailing sadness.

Used in a neutral sense, the term 'coping' refers to one's ability to appraise and respond to a stressful situation. Social support refers to the perceived availability of social support networks.

In the first section of this chapter the measurement of psychosocial well-being will be addressed and this is followed by an examination of the clinical relationship between psychosocial factors and common gastrointestinal conditions, with particular emphasis on inflammatory bowel disease and irritable bowel syndrome. The role of the nurse in the management of psychosocial problems will conclude the chapter.

Measurement of psychological well-being in gastrointestinal medicine

The measurement of psychological morbidity is based on assessment of signs and symptoms of 'dysfunction'. There are numerous scales of psychological well-being, as summarised in Box 13.1.

These scales have been used to measure psychological and psychiatric morbidity in both inflammatory bowel disease and irritable bowel syndrome. The HDS is inappropriate for use in this patient population due to its emphasis on physical symptoms and the high number of items that concern somatic problems. The BDI has high validity and reliability but has been used predominantly in psychiatric populations and is dependent on subjects' ability to accurately report their emotional state. The HAD scale is widely used in clinical trials for a wide range of conditions, including arthritis, cancer, bowel disorders and dental phobias. The tool of choice for nurses measuring psychological well-being in patients with gastrointestinal illnesses is HAD, as it is short and easy to administer and analyse.

Box 13.1   Psychological/psychiatric measurement tools.

Hamilton Depression Scale (HDS)
Beck Depression Inventory (BDI)
Hospital Anxiety and Depression Scale (HAD)

Inflammatory bowel disease

Inflammatory bowel disease (IBD) is reviewed in Chapter 6. It is well recognised that psychosocial factors play a major role in the morbidity of Crohn's disease and ulcerative colitis. Increasing attention is now paid to the patient's subjective views of well-being, including emotional and psychosocial assessment, to provide an holistic measure of disease severity. To evaluate the effect of psychosocial factors on symptoms in IBD it is essential to examine the illness in terms of health-related quality of life (HRQoL). HRQoL differs from objective disease measurement in that it evaluates the patient's perception, beliefs, experience, and function as related to an illness or condition. It incorporates disease-related factors with sociocultural and psychosocial factors. A review of HRQoL assessment is provided in Chapter 14.

Historical perspective of psychological influences in IBD

Crohn made several links between psychological variables and Crohn's disease. Since the first recognition of Crohn's disease in the 1930s, gastroenterologists, surgeons, psychologists and psychiatrists have striven to find a relationship between psychological variables and physical symptoms. This link has been examined in four ways:

(1)   personality associations
(2)   psychopathology in IBD
(3)   relationship with interpersonal factors
(4)   stressful life events leading to onset and exacerbation of IBD

Personality associations in IBD

The earliest psychoanalytically orientated psychosomatic studies conducted in the 1950s described distinct personality traits linked to IBD. The principal proponent of this psychosomatic hypothesis during this period, George Engel, believed that patients with IBD have a symbiotic relationship with their mother, mother-substitute, or an individual on whom they are emotionally dependent. Interest in such psychosomatic models ebbed in the 1960s and they are now discredited because the studies upon which they were developed were found to be methodologically flawed and were subject to investigator bias.

Certain personality traits have been shown to be present in patients with IBD. For example, Crohn's disease sufferers were viewed as constantly wishing to 'be rid of ' events in their lives and were described as 'obsessive compulsive' in nature and in a state of dependency. Personality traits such as repressed rage, suppression of feelings and anxiety are closely associated with Crohn's disease. These early psychological studies in IBD must be viewed with caution; many of the described personality traits are common in any chronic physical illness and are probably not specific to IBD.

Psychopathology in IBD

Using validated criteria produced by the American Psychiatric Association, it has been shown that patients with Crohn's disease have a high prevalence of psychiatric conditions but there is no association between the degree of physical morbidity and the presence of psychiatric disorders. The prevalence of psychiatric illness is similar in ulcerative colitis and non-ulcerative colitis, with no evidence of an association between psychiatric illness and physical morbidity.

There are limited links between physical morbidity and psychiatric illness in ulcerative colitis. In contrast, patients with Crohn's disease have been shown to have a significantly increased incidence of psychopathy and a clear association between the presence of psychiatric illness and degree of physical morbidity (Helzer *et al.* 1984).

One-third of studies undertaken have shown that Crohn's disease causes significant psychiatric morbidity. Affective symptoms, such as anxiety, predominated. Most studies indicate that psychiatric and psychosocial morbidity increase with chronicity and severity in Crohn's disease.

Relationships with interpersonal factors in IBD

Sources of anxiety in IBD patients include concern about surgery, lethargy, perceptions of body-image and hygiene. These concerns may have a significant influence on an individual's psychological health. Patients with ulcerative colitis and Crohn's disease have different worries. Crohn's disease patients appear more concerned with the impact of their disease upon lifestyle, whereas ulcerative colitis patients more commonly report fears of cancer.

In addition, several psychosocial factors are known to modulate the effects of stress on an individual's response to disease. These include self-confidence, self-reliance and an adequate stable social support system.

Research into sexual adjustment in IBD has been mainly restricted to the consequences of surgery and largely remains a taboo area which is rarely discussed openly. The majority of patients adapt well to their surgery but a minority attribute marital tension, unhappiness or even separation to the presence of a stoma.

In terms of educational attainment and employment prospects, IBD patients may lose time from their studies due to their disease, but this does not appear to affect their academic achievements, as measured by exam success. Many more Crohn's disease patients, compared to healthy controls, experience long spells of unemployment, although relatively few lose their job because of their disease. Many patients actively concealed their illness from their employer because it has been shown that employers can practise discrimination against IBD patients. Some patients say that their disease may have contributed to failure to achieve promotion and impaired career development.

Stressful life events leading to onset of IBD

The term 'stress' has many connotations and definitions based on a variety of perspectives of the human condition. It has been defined as 'a state of anxiety produced when events and responsibilities exceed one's coping abilities'.

The link between stress and disease was examined by Hans Seyle (1976), who described the 'general adaptation syndrome'. Seyle defined stress as the non-specific psychobiological responses of the body to any demand placed upon it to adapt. He observed that whether a situation was perceived positively or negatively, the body's physiological response or arousal was similar; he argued that one cannot discriminate between 'good' and 'bad' stress. The 'general adaptation syndrome' is the process by which the body tries to accommodate stress by adapting to it in a three-stage process.

The three stages comprise:

Stage 1: Alarm reaction. The alarm reaction describes a 'fight or flight' response. In this stage several physiological responses occur. Initially this involves the nervous and the endocrine systems, followed by cardiovascular, pulmonary and musculoskeletal responses.

Stage 2: Stage of resistance. The body tries to revert back to a state of physiological calmness, or homeostasis. Because the perception of a threat still exists, however, complete homeostasis is never reached. Instead, the body stays activated or aroused, usually at a lesser intensity than during the alarm but enough to cause a higher metabolic rate in some organs.

Stage 3: Stage of exhaustion. Exhaustion occurs when one (or more) of the organs targeted by specific metabolic processes can no longer meet the demands placed upon it. In its most extreme form this may lead to organ failure and death.

Seyle's general adaptation syndrome outlined the physiological consequences of stress and he identified the pituitary–adrenocortical axis as the major central neuroendocrine mediator of the stress response. Through activation of the hypothalamus there is stimulation of the pituitary gland, which is responsible for secreting several hormones. Adrenocorticotrophic hormone (ACTH) is the most significant in this context, as it stimulates the release of corticosteroids. This results in a variety of physiological effects; the most important is response to physical and psychological stress. Other effects include stimulation of gluconeogenesis in the liver, inhibition of glucose uptake by peripheral tissues and suppression of the immune system, which may be related to IBD.

The relationship between stress and disease involves several factors. These include the cognitive perceptions of the threatening stimuli and the consequent activation of the nervous, endocrine and immune systems.

It has been suggested that psychosocial disruption may contribute to disease susceptibility in IBD. For example, the stress of moving from a nomadic life to government housing may have contributed to the first reported occurrence of ulcerative colitis in Bedouin Arabs, a group in which ulcerative colitis is otherwise extremely rare.

Physiological consequences of stress on the gastrointestinal tract
All clinical gastroenterologists are aware that psychological stress may trigger IBD relapse and it often causes gastrointestinal symptoms. Diarrhoea and abdominal cramps are experienced by most individuals during times of stress, for example prior to an exam or interview.

There are many factors, including emotion, that affect gastrointestinal secretion and motility. These may exert their effects via the central nervous system and produce long-term sensitisation of pathways involved in the transmission of visceral sensation. Several neurotransmitters (e.g. acetylcholine) and hormones (e.g. cholecystokinin) are common to both the gastrointestinal tract and central nervous system (CNS).

Drossman (1993) suggested that prolonged exposure to psychological stress can lead to transient changes in immunological function. He argued that IBD could result from dysregulation of the relationship between the CNS and the immunological function of the gastrointestinal tract. Although psychosocial factors may not initiate inflammation in IBD, he suggested that they may lead to an abnormal immune response, which affects disease activity.

Stress, personality and coping in IBD

Two main approaches to the study of stress in IBD are described here. One line of investigation has examined the causal relationship between stress and disease and the other has examined the effects of relieving stress upon disease activity.

Stress and causation
One way of relating stress to illness has been to link it to life events. The Social Readjustment Rating Scale (SRRS) is an inventory which ranks 43 stressful events with numeric values, from most to least stressful, based upon their capacity to disrupt activities and the degree of readjustment which is necessary following the event. These values are termed 'Life Change Units' (LCU). In further research using this assessment tool, Rahe (1968) demonstrated that the development of minor illnesses, such as colds and 'flu, was linked to life events.

Personality and stress in IBD
Personality has been classified by psychologists as either 'stress-prone' or 'stress-resistant' and individuals with these different characteristics may react very differently to similar stressful events. Type-A, co-dependency and helpless–hopeless are three personality sub-types that have been defined as being stress-prone.

The Type-A Behaviour Pattern (TABP) is characterised by striving for achievement, competitiveness and impatience. TABP may predispose to the development of ischaemic heart disease. However, there is uncertainty over the existence of TABP.

Another influential factor in modulating the stress response is 'locus of control'. This concept arose from the observation that individuals give different reasons for events; the cause of an event could be external (luck), internal (ability and effort) or a combination of the two (Rotter 1966). A person with an internal locus of control has an expectation that he or she will be able to control the environment, either through ability or effort. Someone with an external locus of control expectation believes that outcomes are outside personal control and depend on outside influences. Locus of control has been implicated in a wide range of health-related behaviours, with 'internals' more likely to take a variety of preventive measures than 'externals'. Personal control may modulate affective disturbance and job-strain. A sense of personal control over the environment is one of the principal components of the 'hardy' personality – who in the face of disaster appears immune to stress. Research on 'hardiness' suggested that having more internal control or an internal locus of control may serve as a buffer against stress. However, an internal locus of control has been shown to be associated with a greater susceptibility to stress among subjects who experienced high levels of life events.

Coping in IBD

Coping is a critical factor in adaptation to stressful life events. In this instance 'coping' refers to the ability to appraise and respond to IBD and its management. Folkman and Lazarus (1991) defined coping as 'cognitive and behavioural efforts to manage specific external and/or internal demands that are appraised as taxing or exceeding the resources of the person'. In order for a cognitive process to be considered coping it must involve a purposeful effort. They advocated that 'the best coping is that which changes the person–environment relationship for the better'.

Coping styles may be involved in the response to stress and may be influenced by personality. Some researchers have speculated that the effect of a stressor may be buffered by an appropriate coping mechanism, and to an extent this view reflects popular belief. The supposed benefits of a 'good cry', or for that matter a 'good laugh', are well known but it is less well understood what precisely constitutes an appropriate coping mechanism, and more importantly how to measure such a phenomenon.

Stress, life events and disease activity in IBD

It seems reasonable to expect that relatively trivial daily stressors, which occur as part of everyday life, have lesser effects upon symptoms than do major life events, such as bereavement or divorce. Nevertheless, daily stressors, such as oversleeping, missing the bus or a phone incessantly ringing account for a larger percentage of total stress than major life events. It has been demonstrated that 'stress-exposed' patients demonstrated greater risk of disease relapse than 'unexposed patients'.

There is an association between daily life stress events and disease activity. The effect of major life events rather than minor events is difficult to ascertain. Major life events tend to occur less frequently in most 'normal' individuals than in IBD patients, and longitudinal studies need to be undertaken to address this.

Clinical nurse specialists in IBD

Clinical nurse specialists in IBD are valuable and cost-effective members of gastroenterology teams. IBD nurse specialists have well-defined roles in delivering clinical care, such as specialised care, medication monitoring, patient education and psychological support. Research undertaken to date on IBD clinical nurse specialists has been very general in its nature and there is limited evidence to highlight the specific benefits that an IBD nurse specialist may have upon specific sub-groups of IBD patients (i.e. patients with stoma, patients on specific medications such as methotrexate or infliximab, or patients who receive nurse counselling). The chronicity of IBD and the effects of treatments (surgical and medical) have an impact on the daily life of IBD patients and therefore must influence health-related quality of life (HRQoL). Chapter 14 highlights impaired quality of life in patients with IBD. Patients with Crohn's disease appear more affected by their disease in terms of HRQoL than those with ulcerative colitis (Smith *et al.* 2002).

Irritable bowel syndrome

Irritable bowel syndrome (IBS) is one of the most common gastrointestinal disorders in medical practice and can account for approximately 50% of referrals to gastroenterology outpatient clinics. Between 10 and 15% of the general population may have IBS and it affects females more than males. However, it is estimated that only 10% of people with irritable bowel syndrome seek medical advice and most of those who do are managed in primary care. Those who do consult report more severe gastrointestinal symptoms and an increased level of psychological disturbance compared with those who do not consult. Therefore, pain severity as well as psychological distress may in part explain healthcare seeking.

A clear relationship has been established between psychiatric illness, psychosocial morbidity and IBS in patients who seek medical help. There is, however, some difficulty in interpreting the implications of the comorbidity between IBS and psychiatric disorders such as anxiety and depression. For example, although anxiety, via the autonomic nervous system, has direct effects upon the gastrointestinal tract and may lead to exacerbation of pain, it is also reasonable to suggest that the symptom of abdominal pain in itself may lead to increased feelings of anxiety. Thus, anxiety may be a cause or a consequence of the symptoms of IBS.

An understanding of the role of psychosocial factors is required in IBS in order to optimise patients' care. Drossman (1993) and Thompson (1999) have emphasised the importance of psychosocial treatments in the management of IBS. Psychological treatments including psychotherapy, hypnotherapy, biofeedback, cognitive behavioural therapy and relaxation therapy have been suggested for use in the management of IBS.

Epidemiology of psychosocial factors associated with IBS

There is a strong association between life stressors and IBS. Severe life events or chronic social difficulties, such as bereavement and marital separation, are more frequent in functional bowel disorders than in organic gastrointestinal disorders.

IBS is closely associated with high levels of psychological morbidity. Psychiatric diagnosis often precedes the onset of IBS symptoms. The most common disorders associated with IBS are anxiety and depression.

Relationship between psychosocial factors and physiology in IBS

Psychosocial factors and physiology, principally gut motility and sensation, interact jointly via the central and enteric nervous system. Psychosocial stressors affect colonic motility and this dysmotility may also affect psychological state.

Given the effect of psychosocial factors on the development and course of IBS, it is important to examine the role of psychological therapies in the management of IBS.

Relaxation in IBS

Relaxation provides perhaps the most common and the simplest form of psychotherapy which can be easily taught to patients by nurses. The rationale behind relaxation is that if stress is a factor in the aetiology of IBS, then reducing the emotional tension with relaxation techniques will help to reduce physical symptoms and induce a sense of well-being by allowing the patient to feel more in control. Relaxation therapy normally incorporates some, if not all, of the following elements: lying or sitting in a comfortable position, use of peaceful music, closing eyes to reduce visual stimulation, exercises to relax muscles and visual imagery to elicit peaceful situations. Relaxation therapy is a central component in many multi-component psychotherapeutic regimes used to treat IBS.

Psychological treatments

Although psychological factors do not cause IBS, it is clear that they do influence the natural history of the disease, and psychological therapy may modify disease activity. Treatments include:

- tutorial therapy
- non-specific hypnotic relaxation
- gut-directed hypnotherapy
- nurse-led counselling
- cognitive behavioural therapy

It has been suggested that patients with IBS may benefit from the provision of counselling support, which enables them to cope with their illness and improve HRQoL. A trained IBS nurse counsellor can influence how well patients accept and understand their illness.

In the examination of studies undertaken to determine the impact of psychological treatments in IBS there are many positive findings, which have emerged to warrant a strong case for psychological treatment in IBS. In conclusion, there is a strong suggestion of an association between psychopathology, stressful life events, personality and IBD. Extension of nursing roles has seen the development of many nurse practitioners in IBS to help deal with this psychosocial morbidity.

Hypnotherapy
Hypnotherapy is an altered state of consciousness in which the subject acts only on external suggestion. Consciousness is not lost in hypnosis; it simply becomes more selective and it has been found to be effective for a variety of problems that hinge on emotions, habits, and even the body's involuntary responses. It has been applied to a variety of medical conditions and has been demonstrated to be effective in the treatment of anxiety, tension, depression, phobias and compulsions.

Gut-directed hypnotherapy involves the induction of a trance-like state of deep relaxation by the therapist using techniques of imagery, progressive muscular relaxation and a slow, repetitive, vocal cadence. The establishment of an altered state of consciousness renders the patient susceptible to the therapist's suggestion. Gut-directed hypnotherapy specifically involves bowel-directed imagery to modify gut function.

Gut-directed hypnotherapy involves an overview of smooth muscle physiology in the gut. Patients are then given a short lesson on the basic anatomy and physiology of the gut and this is related to an explanation of the symptoms of IBS. Hypnosis is then induced by an eye fixation technique. Once in a trance state, hypnotised patients are fully aware of their surroundings and are in control of their actions. This altered state of consciousness renders the patient susceptible to the therapist's suggestion. Relaxation techniques, which are related to induction of a reduced state of arousal, are also involved. Once the patient is in a relaxed state it is expected that symptoms and physiological changes that are associated with an exaggerated state of autonomic arousal will disappear.

Visualisation techniques are also used whereby patients are encouraged to imagine the gut as a river. For example, if the patient has diarrhoea they are asked to imagine their bowel as a turbulent stream; the therapist then implants the appropriate imagery to slow it down. During the therapy patients are encouraged to place their hands on their abdomen. The therapist implants the suggestion of a feeling of warmth in the patient's hands; this warm sensation is transferred to their abdomen and the patient is urged to feel the warmth within the muscular lining of their gut to induce relaxation and remove tension.

A final part of this therapy involves ego-strengthening. This is a fundamental requirement to deal with the psychological consequences of an illness, such as anxiety, fear, tension and agitation. Ego-strengthening techniques are used in combination with suggestions of symptom relief to enable the patient to become more self-reliant, more confident and more able to adjust to his or her environment, and thus less prone to symptomatic relapse.

Patients are also taught self-hypnosis at an early stage of the treatment and are provided with audiotapes to encourage this practice at home.

Biofeedback
Biofeedback is another psychotherapeutic technique, used by specialist nurses. It is a behavioural technique of managing gastrointestinal dysfunction and assumes a link between specific physiological response and particular disorders. Biofeedback has been particularly useful in the treatment of bowel disorders, such as diarrhoea, constipation and faecal incontinence. It can be spectacularly effective in such patients, and the possibility that it works by suggestion, harnessing and amplifying the patient's capacity to cure himself does not in any way detract from its effectiveness.

Cognitive behavioural therapy
Cognitive behavioural therapy (CBT) gives patients control over their symptoms through the implicit assumption that their IBS symptoms are related to the abnormal, which the patient can rectify without consultation to a nurse or doctor. CBT is based on the assumption that IBS is a behavioural disease, generated by responses to stressful life events. The nurse who practises CBT will insist that the patient takes responsibility for their illness and helps them find a more healthy way of dealing with the underlying problem.

Conclusion

The psychosocial aspects of gastrointestinal disorders, especially inflammatory bowel disease, are an area where nursing care is of the utmost importance. Inflammatory bowel disorders are poorly understood in terms of aetiology and are especially resistant to treatment. In addition, they have a profound effect on the psychological state of the patient and on quality of life. Where patients lack an explanation of their condition, and medical and surgical intervention can only offer temporary relief, at best, good nursing care can help patients to cope with the adverse effects of the disease and to adhere to treatments which will help reduce their symptoms, even if total relief is elusive.

Nurses can provide general care, in terms of clear and sympathetic explanations of what a patient with inflammatory bowel disease can expect: signs, symptoms and the chronic nature of the condition. Symptoms such as frequency and urgency with diarrhoea are inconvenient and embarrassing; advice about diet and avoiding situations and foods which might stimulate diarrhoea or cause bloating can be invaluable. Simple advice about making sure that toilet facilities are available may seem obvious to the nurse but may be required by the patient. Beyond such essential aspects of nursing care the role of the nurse is expanding into therapies such as counselling which can prove effective in helping some patients to cope with their disease and improve their psychological state and quality of life. Patients with inflammatory bowel disease will have a long-term relationship with medical and nursing services. The role that nurses can play is one which may help patients to get the best out of these services.

REFERENCES

Drossman, D.A. (1993) Psycho-social and psycho-physiologic mechanisms in GI illness. In: *The Growth of Gastroenterologic Knowledge During the 20th Century* (Krisner, J.B., ed.), pp. 419–20. Lea and Febiger, Philadelphia.

Folkman, S. and Lazarus, R.S. (1991) Coping and emotion. In: *Stress and Coping: An Anthology* (Monat, A. and Lazarus, R.S., eds). Columbia University Press, New York.

Helzer, J.E., Channos, S., Norland, C.C., Stillings, W.A. and Alpers, D.H. (1984) A study of the association between Crohn's disease and psychiatric diagnosis. *Gastroenterology*, **86**, 324–5.

Rahe, R.H. (1968) Life change measurement as a predictor of illness. *Proceedings of the Royal Society of Medicine*, **61**, 1124–6.

Rotter, J.B. (1966) Generalised expectancies for internal versus external control of reinforcement. *Psychological Monographs*, **80**, 1–28.

Seyle, H. (1976) *The Stress of Life*. McGraw-Hill, New York.

Smith, G.D., Watson, R., Roger, D., McRorie, E. and Palmer, K.R. (2002) Impact of a nurse-led counselling service on quality of life in patients with inflammatory bowel disease. *Journal of Advanced Nursing*, **38**(2), 152–60.

Thompson, W.G. (1999) Irritable bowel syndrome: a management strategy. *Clinical Gastroenterology*, **13**, 443–60.

Chapter 14
Quality of Life in Gastroenterology

Chapter objectives

After reading this chapter you should understand:

- The concept of health-related quality of life (HRQoL).
- Types of HRQoL measurement tools available.
- HRQoL instruments used in gastrointestinal medicine.

Introduction

In recent years the concept of quality of life has emerged as an area of increasing interest in both nursing and medical care. One of the reasons for the development of this interest in the healthcare setting relates to the growing recognition of the need to understand the impact of disease on patients' lives rather than just upon their bodies. This is particularly important for chronic diseases such as cancer, chronic pain syndromes and chronic inflammatory diseases. Health-related quality of life is a concept that has developed from the need to understand the impact of such diseases. It reflects the physical, social and emotional attitudes and behaviours of an individual as these relate to their previous and current health states. Health-related quality of life assessment describes health status from the patients' perspective and as such can be used as an effective tool to assess and explain disease outcomes.

Research on quality of life in the area of gastroenterology has focused primarily upon chronic gastrointestinal disorders, such as gastro-oesophageal reflux disease (GORD), non-ulcer dyspepsia, inflammatory bowel disease, irritable bowel syndrome and cancer of the gastrointestinal tract.

In this chapter, issues associated with quality of life in relation to gastrointestinal medicine will be examined; these issues are extremely relevant to all nurses who provide care for patients with gastrointestinal disorders.

Understanding the health-related problems of patients will allow nurses to gain increased insight into the nature of the condition and so may help them plan interventions which enhance the well-being of patients. A nurse who is skilled and competent in the management of patients can influence how well these patients accept and understand their illness. The responsibility of the nurse providing care for patients with gastrointestinal disorders has several facets including:

- Obtaining a thorough physical and psychosocial history.
- Formulating a nursing diagnosis with appropriate nursing interventions.
- Teaching patients about their disease and treatments.
- Providing a supportive environment to reduce stress and anxiety.
- Helping to promote a positive self-image.
- Encouraging the teaching of adaptive coping strategies.

In gastroenterology, patients may wait for considerable periods of time for the results of invasive medical diagnostic tests and this waiting may be a difficult, anxious period. Nursing staff have a role in offering support, comfort and reassurance. Specially trained nursing staff will be able to identify and support specific psychological problems associated with gastrointestinal disorders. Nursing care may be enhanced with a good knowledge of health-related quality-of-life issues that are associated with these conditions.

Quality of life

Quality of life (QoL) means so many different things to so many people that its usefulness as a meaningful descriptor is seriously compromised. QoL is a vague term, the origin of which is unknown, but it portrays the essence of attitudes and behaviours in the physical, social and emotional domains of lifestyle. Shin and Johnson (1978) defined QoL as 'the possession of the resources necessary to the satisfaction of individual needs, wants and desires, participation in activities enabling personal development and self actualisation and satisfactory comparison between oneself and others'.

Furthermore, only part of QoL is a consequence of physical health status. McGee *et al.* (1991) questioned patients at a follow-up gastrointestinal outpatient clinic to ascertain the relative importance of a range of aspirations and they concluded that family, work, social, leisure and health were the most frequently nominated.

Significant advances in medical and surgical practice have led to prolonged life but in many patients this may be at the expense of undergoing mutilating surgery or the unpleasant side-effects of drug therapy. Consequently health professionals have become aware that QoL is at least as important as the duration of survival in the provision of health care.

Health-related quality of life: an overview

The theoretical framework of health-related quality of life (HRQoL) is largely based on a multi-dimensional perspective of health based upon a combination of physical, psychological and social well-being. The physical dimension is concerned with the effects of illness on a person's ability to carry out normal activities of daily living. The psychosocial dimensions deal with the effects of illness upon emotion and social interaction with friends, family, work colleagues and the community. Often some psychosocial elements are more important than physical symptoms in patients suffering from chronic illness.

There are five inherent dimensions in HRQoL:

- physical health
- mental health
- social functioning
- role functioning
- general well-being

The most comprehensive definition of HRQoL is provided by the World Health Organisation Quality of Life Group (WHOQOL 1995), which provided a definition including individual perceptions and relationships with the environment:

> 'Quality of life is defined as an individual's perception of their position in life in the context of the culture and value systems in which they live and in relation to their goals, expectations, standards and concerns. It is a broad ranging concept, affected in a complex way by the person's physical health, psychological state, level of independence, social relationships, and their relationships to salient features of the environment.'

This distinguishes HRQoL from other forms of QoL assessment as patient-reported subjective assessments evaluating:

- sensory function (including pain and discomfort)
- mobility
- activities of daily living
- physical function
- social function
- emotional function
- cognitive function

Health and disease-related attitudes and satisfaction are also important components of HRQoL.

Measurement of HRQoL

Health-related quality-of-life measures have several potential uses in aiding routine clinical practice. These are summarised in Box 14.1.

Box 14.1   The value of quality-of-life measures in clinical practice.

- To prioritise problems
- To identify patient preferences
- To facilitate communication
- To screen for potential problems
- To monitor changes or response to treatments
- To train new staff

Other plausible applications of HRQoL measurement within health care involve audit, clinical governance, therapeutic efficacy in clinical trials and as an essential constituent of cost–benefit estimation.

HRQoL measurement is becoming increasingly recognised as an important outcome and predictor for patients with all chronic diseases. HRQoL is generally assessed by patient-completed quantitative questionnaire, which assesses both physical and psychosocial attitudes and function.

There are several key areas which require specific attention when addressing the issue of HRQoL and these are examined below.

Who should measure HRQoL?

Whether HRQoL should be assessed by the patient or by a health professional remains controversial. Many clinicians believe that their own observations are more useful than the patient's views as they provide an objective perspective. However, the subjective view of the patient's own well-being is important and should be viewed as a reliable index of health status. Bowling (1991) reported consensus among health researchers who believed that health outcome should incorporate the patients' perspective, not simply in terms of whether or not a treatment or therapy is successful, but more globally in relation to the patient's perceived mental and physical well-being.

Types of HRQoL measurement

Three main types of HRQoL measures are used in research and practice within gastroenterology: global assessment, generic instruments and disease-specific measures.

Global assessment

The global assessment, usually a graded summary such as 'good', 'fair' or 'poor' or a 10 cm visual analogue scale, may help to predict a relationship between simple parameters such as disease severity and function, but it is often inadequate for more sophisticated hypothesis testing. To outline this, global questions such as, 'How do you rate your quality of life today?' are of limited value. They categorise patients but do not explain why a patient is placed in a particular category. Global measures are nevertheless important in that they do provide constructs against which subjective measures may be validated.

Generic instruments

Generic instruments are also called 'general health status measures'. Generic instruments are multi-item problem lists that are meant to be independent of sex, age and disease. Items are frequently clustered in subscores, such as 'physical' or 'emotional function', 'somatic sensation' or 'mental health', which all appear relevant in IBD. In some instruments these sub-scales may be summarised into one single score.

Garratt *et al.* (1993) illustrated the controversy as to whether or not generic and/or disease-specific measures should be used in the assessment of HRQoL in specific conditions, such as IBD. The main clinical value of generic instruments may be as a supplement to disease-specific tools in the detection of clinical changes.

Generic instruments are measures which implicitly or explicitly aim to gauge broad measures of health status and they have been used in patients with gastroenterology. They include the Sickness Impact Profile (Bergner *et al.* 1981) and the SF-36 (Brazier *et al.* 1992). These questionnaires have been developed to cover specific components of HRQoL in a systematic and unified manner. They are of most value for assessing the multiple medical or severe diseases occurring in older or disabled people. They are also of use in the evaluation of conditions which lack objective end points, such as GORD and irritable bowel syndrome. Generic measures have clinical value because they may reveal symptoms or restrictions of activities that physicians do not elicit from patients.

Summary of generic instruments

Generic scales implicitly or explicitly aim to measure HRQoL. They have evolved in order to make comparisons between varying conditions, to broaden outcome indicators and because of the slow development of disease-specific questionnaires. Until recently, generic assessments represented the predominant method of measuring HRQoL in gastroenterology. Instruments such as SIP and SF-36 are the most commonly used and allow for a direct comparison to be made between individuals or populations with different diseases.

The main constraint of all generic scales is their inability to identify condition-specific aspects of disease. Of the generic measures covered in relation to gastroenterology, the unsatisfactory length of the SIP confirms the SF-36 as the most appropriate generic test for measurement of HRQoL. The SF-36 is internally consistent and provides a valid measure of the health status across a wide range of patients.

Disease-specific measures in gastroenterology

Disease-specific instruments are designed for patients with a particular disease, to identify the most relevant symptoms. Disease-specific tools are usually multi-item inventories that are used to detect important treatment effects or changes in patients with a single condition. Their major disadvantage is that disease-specific scales have not been validated for all known gastrointestinal conditions and some unanticipated problems may be overlooked. To overcome these difficulties it is recommended to use disease-specific questionnaires in combination with generic instruments.

A number of disease-specific questionnaires have been developed to address a range of gastrointestinal disorders, as follows.

Chronic gastrointestinal disorders (GIDs)

The gastrointestinal quality-of-life index was developed to measure HRQoL in multiple GIDs.

HRQoL in GORD

Specific symptoms of GORD, such as heartburn, regurgitation or chest pain, can substantially impair HRQoL. A gastrointestinal symptom rating scale (GSRS) was developed to discriminate between several GIDs (www.qolid.org/public/gsrs accessed 8 May 2004). It contains 15 items and has five domains: abdominal pain syndrome, reflux syndrome, indigestion syndrome, diarrhoea syndrome and constipation syndrome.

The gastro-oesophageal reflux disease health-related quality-of-life scale (GORD-HRQoL) is a ten-item questionnaire developed for surgical patients and at the time of writing requires further assessment. Another questionnaire requiring further psychometric testing is the 12-item heartburn quality of life (HBQoL). These disease-specific instruments can discriminate GORD from other gastrointestinal disorders and stratify patients by symptom severity and are therefore of use in clinical decision making. The GSRS would appear the most robust GORD instrument.

Irritable bowel syndrome

Irritable bowel syndrome (IBS) is characterised by abdominal pain and altered bowel function. The impact of IBS on quality of life has been shown to be clinically significant in patients.

Patients with IBS have difficulty travelling, participating in sport and attending social functions. IBS is an inorganic condition (see Chapter 6) and lack of objective parameters to assess health status has prompted several groups to develop disease-specific measures for IBS.

The 30-item IBSQOL was developed in North America in 1997. It is summed into several dimensions. These are listed in Box 14.2. The current IBSQOL is a 34-item instrument which has been more extensively validated than the previous IBSQOL (Hahn *et al.* 1997). However, further experience with these instruments in the clinical setting is required to determine how best to measure HRQoL in IBS.

Box 14.2   Dimensions of quality of life in IBS.

Emotional health	Mental health
Sleep	Energy/vitality
Physical health	Diet
Social role	Physical role

Inflammatory bowel disease

Inflammatory bowel disease (IBD) has been exposed to extensive evaluation in the HRQoL literature. IBD encompasses both ulcerative colitis and Crohn's disease and is a significant chronic disease affecting primarily young individuals. There is little doubt that inflammatory bowel disease can have a major adverse impact upon many patients' lives. The manifestations of IBD are often severe and affect multiple aspects of a patient's life. Patients with IBD have also been characterised as having psychological problems, such as anxiety and maladaptive coping mechanisms. The disease processes of both Crohn's disease and ulcerative colitis are characterised by cycles of remission and exacerbation of physical symptoms such as altered bowel habit, bowel urgency, abdominal pain, rectal bleeding, weight loss and malnutrition, which in conjunction with psychosocial factors may contribute to overall impairment of quality of life.

Emphasis in care is clearly focused on the control of physical symptoms and disease activity, which are not always the best predictors of overall well-being. Traditional measures of disease activity such as the Crohn's Disease Activity Index (CDAI) (Best *et al.* 1976) and the Harvey–Bradshaw Index (Harvey and Bradshaw 1980), although valid objective measures of intestinal and extraintestinal physical disease activity, do not accurately reflect the impaired quality of life experienced by IBD patients.

Disease-specific instruments are used to detect important treatment effects or changes in disease state with time. Disease-specific tools are also multi-item inventories that have been derived in patients with a single condition.

HRQoL assessment in IBD has been performed using a variety of methods with varying degrees of rigour. Objective markers of disease activity such as the CDAI and the Harvey–Bradshaw Index are largely based upon assessment of physical components of disease and do not include psychological measurements.

The Rating Form of IBD Patient Concerns (RFIPC) is a specialised questionnaire that identifies and prioritises the 25 most important worries and concerns of IBD patients. The RFIPC contains four clinically relevant category scores – disease-related, body-related, inter/intrapersonal and sex-related – which are measured on visual analogue scales (Drossman 1993).

The Inflammatory Bowel Disease Questionnaire (IBDQ) examines four aspects of patients' lives: symptoms directly related to the primary bowel disturbance, systemic effects and emotional and social function (Guyatt *et al.* 1989). The

IBDQ was designed to address areas of function that are important to patients. The questionnaire was designed to be short and simple to administer. Each question contains 7-point Likert scale response categories (relating to frequency, severity and satisfaction) with 7 = 'best function' and 1 = 'worst function'. A Likert scale is a rating system subdivided numerically into a series of ordered responses. Scores are summed to produce a total for each of the four aspects of lifestyle.

Short-form HRQoL measurement scales   The short-form IBDQ (IBDQ-SF) is a five-item questionnaire derived from the entire 32-item questionnaire (Turnbull *et al.* 1996). The IBDQ-SF is a quick and reliable means to measure QOL in IBD. It correlates well with CDAI and provides a useful clinical assessment tool. These shorter scales, which purport to detect meaningful clinical changes in HRQoL in IBD patients, may have an important role to play not only in improving the medical and nursing assessment of IBD patients in the out-patient and community settings but also may permit better management of patients.

Disease-specific HRQoL instruments in IBD have been generated from lists of problems identified by patients. They provide for a useful comparison among similar groups of patients and measure clinically important changes over time. Disease-specific health status measures tend to be more responsive to change than generic measures and their subjectivity allows for identification of the problems that are most bothersome to patients. Of the disease-specific tools covered, the IBDQ has been the most extensively evaluated. Preliminary assessment indicated that the IBDQ is a valid, reliable and responsive measure of therapeutic outcome in the assessment of features of disease not embodied by standard disease activity indices. However, despite these findings it is apparent that further assessment is required for these IBDQ disease-specific measures to allow for critical outcome measures and for evaluation of new therapeutic interventions in IBD. Nursing research should be encouraged to investigate factors which influence psychosocial function in IBD sufferers; more understanding of the psychosocial morbidity may provide nurses with the specific tools/skills to help improve HRQoL in patients. Development and evaluation of new HRQoL instruments in IBD should continue and practitioners should be encouraged to include both generic and disease-specific measures in assessment. There is scope for new HRQoL tools to be developed to assess sub-groups of patients with IBD, with potential sub-scales for Crohn's disease and ulcerative colitis.

Gastrointestinal oncology

Malignancies of the digestive system constitute more than one-fifth of all newly diagnosed cancers. Oesophageal, gastric and colorectal cancer are three of the most common gastrointestinal malignancies, which often do not respond to traditional medical or surgical therapy, necessitating palliative management.

Therefore measurement of HRQoL may be the best outcome measure to assess the success or failure of these treatments and nursing interventions. The European Organisation for Research and Treatment of Cancer core quality-of-life questionnaire (EORTC QOL-C30) was developed for this purpose (Aaronson *et al.* 1993). Symptoms such as nausea, vomiting, pain and fatigue were included in the EORTC-QOL-C30. It should be stressed that this questionnaire is specific for oncology patients; it has not been devised for the specific problems encountered by patients with gastrointestinal malignancies and modification and validation of the core questionnaire.

Conclusion

It is hoped that nurses who care for patients with IBD will gain some benefit from understanding the issues associated with measurement of HRQoL in gastroenterology. The potential applications of HRQoL within medical and nursing practice are far-reaching.

REFERENCES

Aaronson, N.K., Ahmedzai, S. and Bergman, B. (1993) The European Organisation for Research and Treatment of Cancer (QLQ-C30): A quality of life instrument for use in clinical trials in oncology. *Journal of the National Cancer Institute*, **85**, 365–76.

Bergner, N., Bobbitt, R.A. and Carter, W.B. (1981) The sickness impact profile: development and final revision of a health status measure. *Medical Care*, **19**, 787–805.

Best, W.R., Becktel, J.M., Singleton, J.W. and Kam, F. (1976) Development of a Crohn's disease activity index. *Gastroenterology*, **70**, 439–44.

Bowling, A. (1991) The conceptualisation of functioning, health and quality of life. In: *Measuring Health; A review of quality of life measurement scales* (Bowling, A., ed.), pp. 108–9. Open University Press, Buckingham.

Brazier, J.E., Harper, R., Jones, N.M.B., O'Cathain, A., Thomas, K.J., Usherwood, T. *et al.* (1992) Validating the SF-36 health survey questionnaire; new outcome measure for primary care. *British Medical Journal*, **305**, 160–4.

Drossman, D.A. (1993) Psychosocial and psychophysiologic mechanism in GI illness. In: *The Growth of Gastroenterologic Knowledge During the 21st Century* (Krisner, J.B., ed.), pp. 419–20. Lea and Febiger, Philadelphia.

Garratt, A.M., MacDonald, L.M., Ruta, D.A., Russell, I.T., Buckingham, J.K. and Krukowski, Z.H. (1993) Towards the measurement of outcome for patients with varicose veins. *Quality in Health Care*, **2**, 5–10.

Guyatt, G., Mitchell, A., Irvine, E.J., Singer, J., Williams, N., Goodcare, R. and Tompkins, C. (1989) A new measurement of health status for clinical trials in inflammatory bowel disease. *Gastroenterology*, **96**, 804–10.

Hahn, B.A., Kirchdoefer, L.J., Fullerton, S. and Mayer, E. (1997) Evaluation of a new quality of life questionnaire for patients with irritable bowel syndrome. *Alimentary Pharmacology & Therapeutics*, **11**, 547–52.

Harvey, R.G. and Bradshaw, J.M. (1980) A simple index of Crohn's disease activity. *The Lancet*, **1**, 514.

McGee, H.M., O'Boyle, C.A., Hickey, A. *et al.* (1991) Assessing the quality of life of the individual: the SEIQoL with a healthy and gastroenterology unit population. *Psychological Medicine*, **21**, 749–59.

Shin, D.C. and Johnson, D.M. (1978) A vowed happiness as an overall assessment of the quality of life. *Social Indicators Research*, **5**, 475–92.

Turnbull, G.K., Vallis, T.M. and Luyendyk, Y. (1996) The assessment of quality of life in inflammatory bowel disease patients: a five item scale for outpatient use. *Gut*, **39**, A16–A17 (Abstract).

WHOQOL (1995) The World Health Organization Quality of Life assessment: position paper from the World Health Organization. Special issue on Health-Related Quality of Life: what is it and how should we measure it? *Social Science and Medicine*, **41**, 1403–9.

Glossary

achalasia – a motor disorder in which muscles in the lower end of the oesophagus and the lower oesophageal sphincter are unable to relax.

achlorhydria – a lack of hydrochloric acid secretion in gastric juice.

adenocarcinoma – a malignant tumour of glandular epithelium.

aetiology – the study of disease causes.

ampulla of Vater – dilatation formed by the junction of the common bile duct and the pancreatic duct proximal to opening into the duodenum.

anaemia – reduced total blood haemoglobin.

anorexia – lack or loss of appetite for food.

antacid – substance which neutralises gastric acid.

anticholinergic – an agent which blocks parasympathetic nerves.

anti-emetic – drug which prevents or alleviates nausea and vomiting.

antrum – constricted, elongated lower portion of the stomach.

anus – terminal orifice of the gastrointestinal tract.

ascending colon – portion of the large intestine between the caecum and the hepatic flexure.

ascites – the accumulation of serous fluid in the abdominal cavity.

aphagia – inability to swallow.

benign – non-malignant (related to tumours).

bile – greenish-yellow fluid secreted by the liver and deposited into the small intestine via bile ducts.

cardia – portion of stomach that surrounds the gastro-oesophageal region.

chief cells – cells located in the parietal gland of the stomach; secretes pepsinogens.

cholangitis – a bacterial infection of bile in the bile duct.

cholecystectomy – surgical removal of the gall bladder.

cholecystitis – infection in the gall bladder.

cholelithiasis – presence of gallstones.

cholestasis – interruption of bile flow.

cirrhosis – inflammatory disease in the liver.

colectomy – surgical removal of the large bowel.

colitis – inflammatory disease of the colon.

common bile duct – duct formed by the union of the cystic duct and hepatic duct.

computed tomography (CT) – a diagnostic radiographic scanning procedure.

constipation – difficulty in passage of stools or infrequent passage of stools.

Crohn's disease – a chronic inflammatory disease involving any region of the gastrointestinal tract, but most commonly involving the terminal ileum, with thickening of the bowel wall.

deglutition – swallowing.

descending colon – the portion of the colon between the splenic flexure and the sigmoid colon.

diarrhoea – an abnormal increase in stool liquidity and daily stool volume.

diverticulitis – infection in one or more diverticula.

diverticulosis – presence of pouch-like diverticula in the muscular layer of the colon.

dyspepsia – indigestion, usually following meals.

dysphagia – difficulty swallowing.

emetic – substance which causes vomiting.

encephalopathy – disease or degenerative condition of the brain.

endoscopic retrograde pancreatography (ERCP) – a combination of endoscopy and radiography to investigate for pancreatic and biliary disease.

endoscopy – visual examination of a hollow organ with endoscope.

enema – a liquid injected into the rectum.

enteritis – inflammation of the intestines.

epigastric – the upper central abdominal region.

fistula – passage from an internal organ to the body surface or between organs.

gall bladder – pear-shaped organ, acts as a reservoir for bile.

gastrectomy – surgical removal of the stomach.

gastric ulcer – ulcer of the gastric mucosa.

gastro-oesophageal reflux disease (GORD) – relates to the backward flow of stomach contents into the oesophagus.

haemoglobin – oxygen-carrying pigment of red blood cells.

haemorrhoid – a submucosal swelling in the anal canal caused by congestion of veins.

Helicobacter pylori **(HP)** – a Gram-negative micro-organism considered to be implicated in the aetiology of peptic ulcer disease and gastritis.

hepatitis – inflammation of the liver.

hepatocyte – a liver cell.

hepatoma – tumour (primary) of the liver.

histamine$_2$ (H$_2$) blocker – an agent which blocks the receptor site for histamine that is responsible for stimulating gastric secretion.

ileal-caecal valve – a functional valve at the junction of the ileum and the caecum.

ileum – distal portion of the small intestine.

ileus – loss of peristalsis in the small bowel.

irritable bowel syndrome – chronic non-inflammatory bowel disease, characterised by abdominal pain/discomfort, abdominal distension and altered bowel function.

ischaemia – decreased supply of oxygenated blood to an organ.

ischaemic colitis – acute vascular insufficiency of the colon usually involving the portion supplied by the inferior mesenteric artery.

jaundice – yellowish discoloration of skin, mucous membranes and sclera.

jejunum – portion of the small bowel that extends from the duodenum to the ileum.

Lamina propria – connective tissue coat of the mucous membrane.

laxative – an agent that acts to promote the evacuation of the bowel.

lower oesophageal sphincter (cardiac sphincter) – a group of muscles at the distal end of the oesophagus. It regulates the entry of food into the stomach.

malabsorption – relates to impaired intestinal absorption of nutrients.

malignancy – a tumour with the ability to invade and spread to other organs.

Mallory-Weiss tear – a mucosal split at the gastro-oesophageal junction that is usually associated with forceful vomiting.

manometry – the measurement of pressure or contraction, usually in the oesophagus or rectum in gastroenterology.

megacolon – a massively enlarged colon.

metastasis – a process by which tumour cells spread throughout the body.

odynophagia – painful swallowing.

oesophagitis – inflammation of the oesophageal mucosa.

pancreatitis – inflammatory disease of the pancreas.

pancreatic enzyme sufficiency – a deficiency in pancreatic exocrine function which leads to malabsorption of fats and other nutrients.

parenteral – administration of nutrition or medication by an injection route (subcutaneous, intramuscular or intravenous).

parietal cells – acid-secreting cells of the stomach (also known as oxyntic cells).

peptic ulcer – an ulcer of the mucous membrane of the oesophagus, stomach or small bowel, caused by action of acidic gastric juice.

percutaneous endoscopic gastrostomy (PEG) – endoscopic insertion of a gastrostomy feeding tube for enteral feeding.

peristalsis – bands of circular muscle contraction that cause the movement of digestive contents through the gastrointestinal tract.

peritonitis – inflammatory disease of the peritoneum.

Peyer's patch – a concentrated region of lymphoid tissue on the mucosa of the small intestine.

pyloric sphincter – physiological muscular sphincter that controls the passage of food from the stomach into the small intestine.

pylorus – distal region of the stomach.

rectum – distal portion of the colon.

ruga – fold of mucosa of stomach (plural: rugae).

satiety – loss of feeling of hunger.

steatorrhoea – condition with high fat content in faeces.

stoma – an opening established in the abdominal wall by either a colostomy or ileostomy.

stress ulcer – an acute form of gastritis that is related to severe trauma or illness.

ulcerative colitis – chronic, recurrent ulceration of the colon.

upper oesophageal sphincter – physiological sphincter at the upper end of the oesophagus.

varices – dilated veins, can occur in oesophagus or stomach.

Useful Addresses

Local addresses are usually listed in the telephone directory or Yellow Pages under Social Services, Welfare Organisations and Charitable Organisations.

British Colostomy Association
15 Station Road
Reading
Berkshire
RGI 1LG
www.bcass.org.uk
Provides information and support to colostomy patients before and after surgery.

British Liver Trust
Portman House
44 High Street
Ringwood
Hampshire
BH24 1AG
www.britishlivertrust.org.uk
Provides information, support and advice concerning liver disease.

British Society of Gastroenterology
3 St Andrews Place
Regent's Place
London
NW1 4LB
www.bsg.org.uk
Encourages education, training and clinical audit in the field of gastroenterology.

Cancer BACUP
3 Bath Place
Rivington Street
London
EC2A 3JR
www.cancerbacup.org.uk
Provides information and support for cancer patients and relatives using a telephone and written answer service by nurses.

Coeliac Society
P.O. Box 220
High Wycome
Bucks
NG11 2HY
www.coeliac.co.uk
Provides advice and counselling concerning coeliac disease and diet.

Digestive Disorders Foundation
3 St Andrew's Place
Regent's Park
London
NW1 4LB
www.digestivedisorders.org.uk
Produces patient-orientated leaflets and supports research.

Eating Disorders Association
103 Prince of Wales Road
Norwich
NR1 1DW
www.edauk.com
Offers mutual support for eating disorders and promotes sharing of information.

Gastrointestinal Nursing
Nursing Standard House
RCN Publishing
The Heights
59–65 Lowlands Road
Harrow
Middlesex
HA1 3AE
www.nursing-standard.co.uk
Gastrointestinal Nursing *is a journal which seeks to promote professional excellence and encourage creativity in nursing.*

ia (Ileostomy and Internal Pouch Support Group)
Peverill House
1–5 Mill Road
Ballyclare
Co Antrim
BT39 9DR
www.the-ia.org.uk
Provides advice to anyone with an ostomy.

Irritable Bowel Syndrome Network
Northern General Hospital
Sheffield
S5 7AU
www.ibsnetwork.org.uk
An independent self-help organisation run by people with IBS.

Macmillan Cancer Relief
89 Albert Embankment
London
SE1 7UQ
www.macmillan.org.uk
Provides support for nurses. Local numbers appear in the telephone directory.

National Association for Colitis and Crohn's Disease
4 Beaumont House
Sutton Road
St. Albans
Herts
AL1 5HH
www.nacc.org.uk
Offers support and information for patients with IBD and their families.

Nursing services
Health visitors
Community Nurses
District Nurses
Local services listed under 'Nurses' in the telephone directory

Appendix: Nursing & Midwifery Council
Code of Professional Conduct

Code of professional conduct

As a registered nurse, midwife or health visitor, you are personally accountable for your practice. In caring for patients and clients, you must:

- respect the patient or client as an individual
- obtain consent before you give any treatment or care
- protect confidential information
- co-operate with others in the team
- maintain your professional knowledge and competence
- be trustworthy
- act to identify and minimise risk to patients and clients.

These are the shared values of all the United Kingdom healthcare regulatory bodies.

This *Code of professional conduct* was published by the Nursing and Midwifery Council in April 2002 and came into effect on 1 June 2002.

1 Introduction

1.1 The purpose of the *Code of professional conduct* is to:

- inform the professions of the standard of professional conduct required of them in the exercise of their professional accountability and practice
- inform the public, other professions and employers of the standard of professional conduct that they can expect of a registered practitioner.

1.2 As a registered nurse, midwife or health visitor, you must:

- protect and support the health of individual patients and clients
- protect and support the health of the wider community

- act in such a way that justifies the trust and confidence the public have in you
- uphold and enhance the good reputation of the professions.

1.3   You are personally accountable for your practice. This means that you are answerable for your actions and omissions, regardless of advice or directions from another professional.

1.4   You have a duty of care to your patients and clients, who are entitled to receive safe and competent care.

1.5   You must adhere to the laws of the country in which you are practising.

2   As a registered nurse, midwife or health visitor, you must respect the patient or client as an individual

2.1   You must recognise and respect the role of patients and clients as partners in their care and the contribution they can make to it. This involves identifying their preferences regarding care and respecting these within the limits of professional practice, existing legislation, resources and the goals of the therapeutic relationship.

2.2   You are personally accountable for ensuring that you promote and protect the interests and dignity of patients and clients, irrespective of gender, age, race, ability, sexuality, economic status, lifestyle, culture and religious or political beliefs.

2.3   You must, at all times, maintain appropriate professional boundaries in the relationships you have with patients and clients. You must ensure that all aspects of the relationship focus exclusively upon the needs of the patient or client.

2.4   You must promote the interests of patients and clients. This includes helping individuals and groups gain access to health and social care, information and support relevant to their needs.

2.5   You must report to a relevant person or authority, at the earliest possible time, any conscientious objection that may be relevant to your professional practice. You must continue to provide care to the best of your ability until alternative arrangements are implemented.

3   As a registered nurse, midwife or health visitor, you must obtain consent before you give any treatment or care

3.1   All patients and clients have a right to receive information about their condition. You must be sensitive to their needs and respect the wishes of those who refuse or are unable to receive information about their condition. Information should be accurate, truthful and presented in such a way as to make it easily understood. You may need to seek legal or professional advice, or guidance from your employer, in relation to the giving or withholding of consent.

3.2   You must respect patients' and clients' autonomy – their right to decide whether or not to undergo any health care intervention – even where a refusal may result in harm or death to themselves or a foetus, unless a court of law orders to the contrary. This right is protected in law, although in circumstances where the health of the foetus would be severely compromised by any refusal to give consent, it would be appropriate to discuss this matter fully within the team, and possibly to seek external advice and guidance (see clause 4).

3.3   When obtaining valid consent, you must be sure that it is:

- given by a legally competent person
- given voluntarily
- informed.

3.4   You should presume that every patient and client is legally competent unless otherwise assessed by a suitably qualified practitioner. A patient or client who is legally competent can understand and retain treatment information and can use it to make an informed choice.

3.5   Those who are legally competent may give consent in writing, orally or by co-operation. They may also refuse consent. You must ensure that all your discussions and associated decisions relating to obtaining consent are documented in the patient's or client's health care records.

3.6   When patients or clients are no longer legally competent and thus have lost the capacity to consent to or refuse treatment and care, you should try to find out whether they have previously indicated preferences in an advance statement. You must respect any refusal of treatment or care given when they were legally competent, provided that the decision is clearly applicable to the present circumstances and that there is no reason to believe that they have changed their minds. When such a statement is not available, the patients' or clients' wishes, if known, should be taken into account. If these wishes are not known, the criteria for treatment must be that it is in their best interests.

3.7   The principles of obtaining consent apply equally to those people who have a mental illness. Whilst you should be involved in their assessment, it will also be necessary to involve relevant people close to them; this may include a psychiatrist. When patients and clients are detained under statutory powers (mental health acts), you must ensure that you know the circumstances and safeguards needed for providing treatment and care without consent.

3.8   In emergencies where treatment is necessary to preserve life, you may provide care without patients' or clients' consent, if they are unable to give it, provided you can demonstrate that you are acting in their best interests.

3.9   No-one has the right to give consent on behalf of another competent adult. In relation to obtaining consent for a child, the involvement of those with parental responsibility in the consent procedure is usually necessary, but will depend on the age and understanding of the child. If the child is under the age of 16 in England and Wales, 12 in Scotland and 17 in Northern Ireland, you must be aware of legislation and local protocols relating to consent.

3.10   Usually the individual performing a procedure should be the person to obtain the patient's or client's consent. In certain circumstances, you may seek consent on behalf of colleagues if you have been specially trained for that specific area of practice.

3.11   You must ensure that the use of complementary or alternative therapies is safe and in the interests of patients and clients. This must be discussed with the team as part of the therapeutic process and the patient or client must consent to their use.

4   As a registered nurse, midwife or health visitor, you must co-operate with others in the team

4.1   The team includes the patient or client, the patient's or client's family, informal carers and health and social care professionals in the National Health Service, independent and voluntary sectors.

4.2   You are expected to work co-operatively within teams and to respect the skills, expertise and contributions of your colleagues. You must treat them fairly and without discrimination.

4.3   You must communicate effectively and share your knowledge, skill and expertise with other members of the team as required for the benefit of patients and clients.

4.4   Health care records are a tool of communication within the team. You must ensure that the health care record for the patient or client is an accurate account of treatment, care planning and delivery. It should be consecutive, written with the involvement of the patient or client wherever practicable and completed as soon as possible after an event has occurred. It should provide clear evidence of the care planned, the decisions made, the care delivered and the information shared.

4.5   When working as a member of a team, you remain accountable for your professional conduct, any care you provide and any omission on your part.

4.6   You may be expected to delegate care delivery to others who are not registered nurses or midwives. Such delegation must not compromise existing care but must be directed to meeting the needs and serving the interests of patients and clients. You remain accountable for the appropriateness of the delegation, for ensuring that the person who does the work is able to do it and that adequate supervision or support is provided.

4.7   You have a duty to co-operate with internal and external investigations.

5   As a registered nurse, midwife or health visitor, you must protect confidential information

5.1   You must treat information about patients and clients as confidential and use it only for the purposes for which it was given. As it is impractical to obtain consent every time you need to share information with others, you should ensure that patients and clients understand that some information may be made available to other members of the team involved in the delivery of care. You must guard against breaches of confidentiality by protecting information from improper disclosure at all times.

5.2   You should seek patients' and clients' wishes regarding the sharing of information with their family and others. When a patient or client is considered incapable of giving permission, you should consult relevant colleagues.

5.3   If you are required to disclose information outside the team that will have personal consequences for patients or clients, you must obtain their consent. If the patient or client withholds consent, or if consent cannot be obtained for whatever reason, disclosures may be made only where:

- they can be justified in the public interest (usually where disclosure is essential to protect the patient or client or someone else from the risk of significant harm)
- they are required by law or by order of a court.

5.4   Where there is an issue of child protection, you must act at all times in accordance with national and local policies.

6   As a registered nurse, midwife or health visitor, you must maintain your professional knowledge and competence

6.1   You must keep your knowledge and skills up-to-date throughout your working life. In particular, you should take part regularly in learning activities that develop your competence and performance.

6.2   To practise competently, you must possess the knowledge, skills and abilities required for lawful, safe and effective practice without direct supervision. You must acknowledge the limits of your professional competence and only undertake practice and accept responsibilities for those activities in which you are competent.

6.3   If an aspect of practice is beyond your level of competence or outside your area of registration, you must obtain help and supervision from a competent practitioner until you and your employer consider that you have acquired the requisite knowledge and skill.

6.4 You have a duty to facilitate students of nursing and midwifery and others to develop their competence.

6.5 You have a responsibility to deliver care based on current evidence, best practice and, where applicable, validated research when it is available.

7 As a registered nurse, midwife or health visitor, you must be trustworthy

7.1 You must behave in a way that upholds the reputation of the professions. Behaviour that compromises this reputation may call your registration into question even if is not directly connected to your professional practice.

7.2 You must ensure that your registration status is not used in the promotion of commercial products or services, declare any financial or other interests in relevant organisations providing such goods or services and ensure that your professional judgement is not influenced by any commercial considerations.

7.3 When providing advice regarding any product or service relating to your professional role or area of practice, you must be aware of the risk that, on account of your professional title or qualification, you could be perceived by the patient or client as endorsing the product. You should fully explain the advantages and disadvantages of alternative products so that the patient or client can make an informed choice. Where you recommend a specific product, you must ensure that your advice is based on evidence and is not for your own commercial gain.

7.4 You must refuse any gift, favour or hospitality that might be interpreted, now or in the future, as an attempt to obtain preferential consideration.

7.5 You must neither ask for nor accept loans from patients, clients or their relatives and friends.

8 As a registered nurse, midwife or health visitor, you must act to identify and minimise the risk to patients and clients

8.1 You must work with other members of the team to promote health care environments that are conducive to safe, therapeutic and ethical practice.

8.2 You must act quickly to protect patients and clients from risk if you have good reason to believe that you or a colleague, from your own or another profession, may not be fit to practise for reasons of conduct, health or competence. You should be aware of the terms of legislation that offer protection for people who raise concerns about health and safety issues.

8.3   Where you cannot remedy circumstances in the environment of care that could jeopardise standards of practice, you must report them to a senior person with sufficient authority to manage them and also, in the case of midwifery, to the supervisor of midwives. This must be supported by a written record.

8.4   When working as a manager, you have a duty toward patients and clients, colleagues, the wider community and the organisation in which you and your colleagues work. When facing professional dilemmas, your first consideration in all activities must be the interests and safety of patients and clients.

8.5   In an emergency, in or outside the work setting, you have a professional duty to provide care. The care provided would be judged against what could reasonably be expected from someone with your knowledge, skills and abilities when placed in those particular circumstances.

Glossary

Accountable	Responsible for something or to someone.
Care	To provide help or comfort.
Competent	Possessing the skills and abilities required for lawful, safe and effective professional practice without direct supervision.
Patient and client	Any individual or group using a health service.
Reasonable	The case of *Bolam* v. *Friern Hospital Management Committee* (1957) produced the following definition of what is reasonable. 'The test is the standard of the ordinary skilled man exercising and professing to have that special skill. A man need not possess the highest expert skill at the risk of being found negligent . . . it is sufficient if he exercises the skill of an ordinary man exercising that particular art.' This definition is supported and clarified by the case of *Bolitho* v. *City and Hackney Health Authority* (1997).

FURTHER INFORMATION

This *Code of professional conduct* is available on the Nursing and Midwifery Council's website at www.nmc-uk.org. Printed copies can be obtained by writing to the Publications Department, Nursing and Midwifery Council, 23 Portland Place, London W1B 1PZ, by fax on 020 7436 2924 or by e-mail at publications@nmc-uk.org. A wide range of NMC standards and guidance publications expand upon and develop many of the professional issues and themes identified in the *Code of professional conduct*. All are available on the NMC's website. A list of current NMC publications is available either on the website or on request from the Publications Department as above.

Enquiries about the issues addressed in the *Code of professional conduct* should be directed in the first instance to the NMC's professional advice service at the address above, by e-mail at advice@nmc-uk.org, by telephone on 020 7333 6541/6550/6553 or by fax on 020 7333 6538.

The Nursing and Midwifery Council will keep this *Code of professional conduct* under review and any comments, suggestions or requests for further clarification are welcome, both from practitioners and members of the public. These should be addressed to the Director of Policy and Standards, NMC, 23 Portland Place, London W1B 1PZ.

April 2002

Summary

As a registered nurse, midwife or health visitor, you must:

- respect the patient or client as an individual
- obtain consent before you give any treatment or care
- co-operate with others in the team
- protect confidential information
- maintain your professional knowledge and competence
- be trustworthy
- act to identify and minimise the risk to patients and clients

Index